DENTAL SCIENCE, MATERIALS AND TECHNOLOGY

POLYMERIC MATERIALS IN DENTISTRY

DENTAL SCIENCE, MATERIALS AND TECHNOLOGY

Dental Materials Research
Haden D. Kaminski and Easton A. DuPois (Editors)
2009. ISBN: 978-1-60741-104-8

Dental Implantation and Technology
Paul A. Williams (Editor)
2010. ISBN: 978-1-60876-209-5

Polymeric Materials in Dentistry
Irini D. Sideridou
2010. ISBN: 978-1-61668-529-4
2010. ISBN: 978-1-61668-399-3 (E-book)

Psychogenic Denture Intolerance: Theoretical Background, Prevention, and Treatment Possibilities
Tibor Károly Fábián and Pal Fejerdy
2010. ISBN: 978-1-61668-621-5
2010. ISBN: 978-1-61728-239-3 (E-book)

DENTAL SCIENCE, MATERIALS AND TECHNOLOGY

POLYMERIC MATERIALS IN DENTISTRY

IRINI D. SIDERIDOU

Nova Science Publishers, Inc.
New York

LIBRARY OF CONGRESS CATALOGING-IN-PUBLICATION DATA

Polymeric materials in dentistry / Irini D. Sideridou.
p. ; cm.
Includes bibliographical references and index.
ISBN 978-1-61668-529-4 (hardcover)
1. Polymers in dentistry. I. Title.
[DNLM: 1. Dental Materials. 2. Polymers. WU 190 S568p 2010]
RK655.5.S53 2010
617.6'95--dc22

2010003162

Published by Nova Science Publishers, Inc. † New York

CONTENTS

PREFACE

The use of polymers for dental purposes started with Goodyears's invention of vulcanized rubber (Vulcanite) in 1839.Vulcanite and further developed thermoplastic materials were used as denture base material for almost 100 years. In the mid-1930s the development of the dough technique made it possible to use polyacrylates in dentistry. By mixing powder of poly(methyl methacrylate) (PMMA) with the monomer the dough could be polymerized by heat initiation. The physical and mechanical properties of the cured base denture can be optimized by the proper selection of an initiator, plasticizer, pigment and cross-linking agents (di- or trifunctional methacrylates) The developing of the redox initiators for the polymerization of methacrylates at room temperature made possible the direct application of these materials as filling resins.

In 1962 Bowen introduced a new polymer by polymerization of Bis-phenol-A-diglycidylether dimethacrylate (Bis-GMA) with a ceramic filler added. Application of a silane as a coupling agent beteen the two components increased the strength characteristics. These polymer composites have been the subject of considerable academic research and are now used widely in operative dentistry. Polymer composites together with the glass-ionomer cements invented in 1969 and first clinically in the early 1970s have a wider application than any other restorative material available to the dental profession. The introduction of photopolymerization of dental resins in the mid-1970s started a new era in operative dentistry.

This book has been written in an effort to emphasize the use of polymeric materials in dentistry nowadays. The text begins with a chapter describing the history of the use of polymeric materials in restorative dentistry, which is followed by six chapters. Chapter 2 is concerned with the polymeric dental prosthetic materials (denture bases, crown and bridge materials and polymeric cements). Much attention is given to the chemical structure and the physic-chemical properties of these materials. In Chapter 3 the polymeric dental restorative materials (polymeric composites, pit and fissure sealants and adhesives) is discussed. In Chapter 4 the applications of polymers in oral and maxillofacial surgery are reported. In Chapter 5 the applications of polymers in therapy of gingivitis and periodontitis (polymers for controlled drug delivery and guided tissue regeneration) are discussed shortly. In Chapter 6 the applications of polymers in orthodontic treatments are presented and finally in Chapter 7 the polymeric dental impression materials (polysulfides, silicones and polyethers) are discussed. It must be mentioned that much attention is given in Chapter 2 and mainly in Chapter 3 because much research work has been done in our lab on the topics presented in these Chapters.

The aim of this text book is to help the readers to understand the chemical structure of the polymeric materials used nowadays in dentistry and the relationship between the chemical structure of these materials and their properties.

Chapter 1

HISTORICAL OVERVIEW

There are four main groups of widely used materials in dentistry: metals and alloys, ceramics, synthetic organic polymers and biopolymers and composites consisted of a polymeric matrix of different kinds of polymers filled with inorganic fine particles. Although several metallic biomaterials are widely used due to their good properties they show a slow and progressive decrease in specific applications which is concomitant to an increase in the use of polymers, composites and inorganic materials. This might have different explanations such as (a) non-precious metal alloys can be chemically unstable in the oral environment (etching, oxidation, pigmentation); (b) a general negative feeling against visible alloys in dentistry has appeared in recent years based on esthetic criteria; (c) many of the non-precious metal alloys frequently show biological complications (allergenicity, cytotoxicity, carcinogenicity; (d) complex equipment is required for metal processing, which usually makes its dental application too expensive; (e) the price of many metals is not balanced and depends on economic or political crisis. These changes in use tendency are characterized by (a) increased use of polymers, polymer composites, and ceramics; (b) development of new techniques for covering metal surfaces with polymer or ceramic materials; (c) development of composites for specific dental applications and (d) improvement of adhesiveness of all these materials to dental structures [1].

History indicates that use of new types of materials for restorative purposes has often shortly followed the development and introduction of new technology and methods to the scientific world. Prof Frederick Rueggeberg in his excellent review article provides historical background on the development of dental polymer-based materials [2]. The dental community, in its search for better, less expensive, easier-to-handle materials, is often quick to adapt a rising technology for new and different purposes. The use of polymer-based materials in dentistry has risen exponentially. Hardly a single clinical procedure is accomplished without use of one or more of these products, which include sealants, dentin bonding agents, restorative composites, fiber-reinforced polymer materials, cementing and lining agents, denture base materials, denture teeth, denture liners, maxillofacial prosthetic products, core buildup materials, orthodontic appliances, splinting materials, temporary restorative materials, and veneers.

Before synthetic polymer systems were developed, many items classified as “plastic” materials were developed from natural resins or exudates and tissues from plants, animals, and insects. It was found that heating these materials would put them in a softened state, permitting them to be molded and shaped prior to their cooling. The first examples of such materials were horns and hoofs of animals. With respect to insect exudates, the most notable are shellac products, which are still in use today. These materials are derived from resins produced by tiny insects (Coccus Lacca) that infest fig trees: literally Shell Lacca, from whence we derive the word “shellac.” Early use of the product was as a protective coating and decorative finish for wood fillers to provide a moldable substance, and bulk products (primarily decorative cases) were produced. As the photography industry grew, the need for inexpensive yet decorative picture frames increased, and shellac was used to fulfill the need. Later, more durable products such as early phonograph discs and 78-rpm records were made by incorporating mineral filler. Even though this material offered ease of shaping with increased temperature, there is no recorded use of shellac for dental purposes.

An important and well-known plant exudate used in dentistry is gutta-percha also known as Corallite. This product is quite similar in structure to natural rubber, differing only by a cis- or trans-relationship (Fig. 1.1). The difference in configuration between these two molecules is slight and relates to how carbon atoms are attached to the unsaturated carbon-to-carbon double bond: either in-line with cis- (natural rubber) or trans- (gutta-percha) to the polymer chain. This small difference results in large differences in physical properties. In the bulk state, natural rubber is soft and highly flexible, has a low melting point, and is tacky. Conversely, gutta-percha is tough and hard, has a high melting point, and exhibits little flexibility. The important aspect of thermo-plasticity was demonstrated. This property is the ability of a material to be heated, molded to a different shape, and cooled and then retained the new conformation. One popular and successful application of this material in dentistry was as a "stopping material," used for the purpose of providing a temporary filling material in emergency situations. Gutta-percha also was used to manufacture direct, temporary crowns. It was even advocated as a definitive restorative material. Moreover, owing to its easy of molding in confined spaces, the use of gutta-percha as endodontic root canal filler became popular and is still widely used today.

Caoutchouc, a South American Indian word meaning "trees that weep" also referred to as "elastic resin" and "India rubber," was developed in 1735 in France. It is a natural resin exuded from specific trees and has a repetitive polyisoprene structure (Figure 1.1). With use of solvents, natural rubber could be made to adapt to a variety of molded shapes. Its glass transition temperature, however, was quite high (48°F). Below this temperature, natural rubber became a hard, rigid solid; above it, the material was soft and flexible. In 1839, Dr Charles Goodyear, Jr, discovered that a mixture of sulfur with caoutchouc (natural rubber) provided materials with greatly improved properties, thus widening the scope of possible commercial uses for this compound. Rubber flexibility could be retained, but the glass transition temperature was markedly lowered from that of the natural state. Addition of sulfur to natural rubber combined unreacted carbon-to-carbon double bonds in the polyisoprene molecule with sulfur units.

In the process, individual rubber molecule chains were covalently bonded, forming cross-links. The treatment greatly improved elastic characteristics and depending on the frequency of cross-links, provided a wide range in flexibility and hardness to the finished product. This process, known as "vulcanization," is still in use today in the rubber industry, especially in the manufacture of tires. In the 19th century, many household, personal, and industrial items were formulated with vulcanized rubber, which revolutionized the industry. With development of technology for extruding, pressing, and forming materials for shape molding, a wide variety of common-day items were made. In 1851, Nelson Goodyear, Charles' brother, developed and patented a manufacturing process for making hard rubber, which he named *Vulcanite*. Development of this hard form of rubber resulted in a tremendous number of consumer items, one of the most popular being eyeglass frames. In 1853, the first denture base was constructed from Vulcanite. Strips of prepared rubber material were placed into the master mold, against a master cast, and steam-heated under pressure. The resulting denture base, with retained porcelain teeth, thus was formed. With the invention of anesthesia for dental extractions, most dental work in the mid 19th century consisted of extractions and full or partial replacements. Thus, the need for an inexpensive, durable denture base quickly arose. The advantages of Vulcanite were its ease of formability, good adaptation to the master cast, and insolubility and non-reactivity in saliva. Its major drawback was that of color. In the processed state, Vulcanite was a dark brown to gray material. To overcome this color problem, various compounds were used to alter the final coloration. However, the addition of components in amounts necessary to obviate the natural color served to weaken the final properties of Vulcanite. By 1891, use of Vulcanite as a denture base material was considered "universal," but at the turn of the century, dentists still wanted a more esthetic, easily moldable material to use for restorative purposes. A material developed during this time that competed with Vulcanite as a denture base was celluloid. Derived from plant framework, this material had to undergo many processes before being ready for use. The product was prepared as "blanks" that were placed in the master mold, heated, and subjected to pressure to make the material adapt to the model, the retentive features of the denture teeth, and to coalesce the blanks into one cohesive mass. Celluloid was first introduced in 1869, when Vulcanite licensing battles were ongoing. The material provided a less expensive alternative to the high cost of purchasing a Vulcanite license and paying the per-tooth fee. Celluloid had more of a natural gingival color than Vulcanite but was more prone to change in shape over time. Celluloid also tended to turn green with age and developed a bad smell from absorbing salivary components.

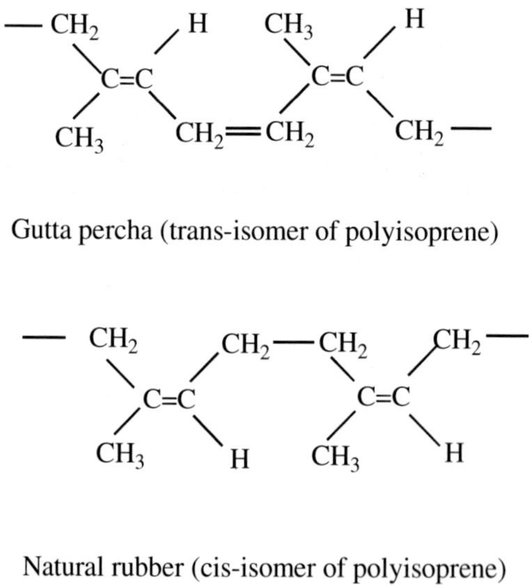

Figure 1.1. Molecular diagrams of A, gutta-percha and B, natural rubber.

A process was developed that provided for a rubber denture base material, a celluloid gum work area and porcelain teeth. This product was known as *New Mode Continuous*, and it offered the best of both worlds at that time: it was flexible, allowed easy fabrication of denture bases, and simulated gingival tissue better than any formulation of Vulcanite. However, the profession still wanted a material of better strength and cosmetic appearance. The following statement, taken from the same late-19th-century textbook cited above, summarizes the feelings of that time (and perhaps epitomizes the timeless wish for easier to use and better materials in dentistry): "Possibly some as yet unknown vulcanizable transparent resin may be found carrying into its combinations enough translucency to give that peculiar, life-like animation which now characterizes porcelain-gum colors."

The period from 1910 to 1950 can be referred to as the age of thermoplastics. Thermoplastic polymers display a physical change with heating, undergoing long-chain, segmental movement and distortion. They may be pressed into a new shape when heated; upon cooling, they will retain that shape. After this period, chemical technology progressed with the introduction of cross-linked polymers, which limit the ability of chains to slip past one another when heated. Thus these materials, the thermoset polymers, are polymerized into shape and not pressed to form. It was during the early 20th century that an embryonic understanding of polymerization developed along with the concept of macromolecules. In 1922, Dr Herman Staudinger, in his work on styrene copolymers, was the first to use the term "macro-molecules" in relationship to polymers. He later received the Nobel Prize in 1953 for his work. It is interesting to note that the definition of the term "plastic" underwent a distinct change in the early 20th century. In 1891, the following definition was presented: "Plastic work includes all dental substitutes in which the base plate is brought into contact with the teeth and the model of pares to be fitted whilst in a fluid, softened, or plastic condition, then hardened, during continuance of this contact, wither by the application or the withdrawal of heat. Plasticity thus used is the property of being molded." Subsequent to 1900, the definition of "plastic" was expanded to include "materials that 'set' or polymerize by chemical reaction or by the evaporation of a solvent." Polymer development after the turn of the century progressed at a staggering pace. Some of the following products, developed during the first three decades of the century, are still used extensively today: cellulose acetate (1903) (Figure 1.2); Bakelite (phenol-formaldehyde, 1907) (Figure 1.3); polystyrene (PS) (1911, 1929), poly(vinyl chloride) (PVC) and poly(vinyl acetate) (1912) (Figure 1.4); Alkyd resins (1914) (Synthetic resins formed by the condensation of polyhydric alcohols with polybasic acids. The most common polyhydric alcohol used is glycerol, and polybasic acid is phthalic anhydride) (Figure 1.5); urea-formaldehyde resins (UF) (1923) (Figure 1.6); polyester (1932) (the term "polyester" as a specific material most commonly refers to polyethylene terephthalate (PET) (Figure 1.7); Melamine-formaldehyde resins (MF) (1933) (Figure 1.8); Nylon (1934) (Nylon is a man-made fiber that makes a good substitute for silk. Wallace Carothers, an organic chemist who was employed at the E.I. du Pont de Nemours & Company, is credited with inventing nylon in 1934.) (Figure 1.9); Low-density polyethylene (LDPE) (1935) (LDPE has a density ranging from 0.91 to 0.93 g/cm^3 (0.60 to 0.61 oz/cu in). The molecules of LDPE have a carbon backbone with side groups of four to six carbon atoms attached randomly along the main backbone. LDPE is the most widely used of all plastics, because it is inexpensive, flexible, extremely tough, and chemical-resistant. LDPE is molded into bottles, garment bags, frozen food packages, and plastic toys); Teflon or poly(tetrafluoro ethylene) (PTFE) (1938) and epoxy resin (1939). The epoxy resins are prepared by condensation reactions of a diepoxide with an amine. The diepoxide usually is the diglycidyl ether of bisphenol A which is the reaction product of bisphenol A with epichlohydrin (Figure 1.10).

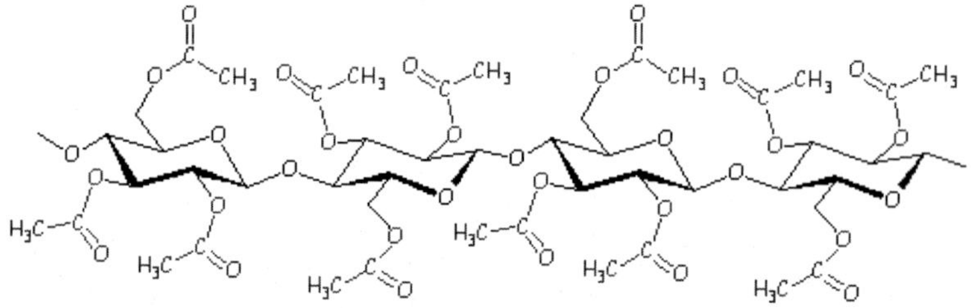

Figure 1.2. Chemical structure of cellulose acetate (or cellulose triacetate).

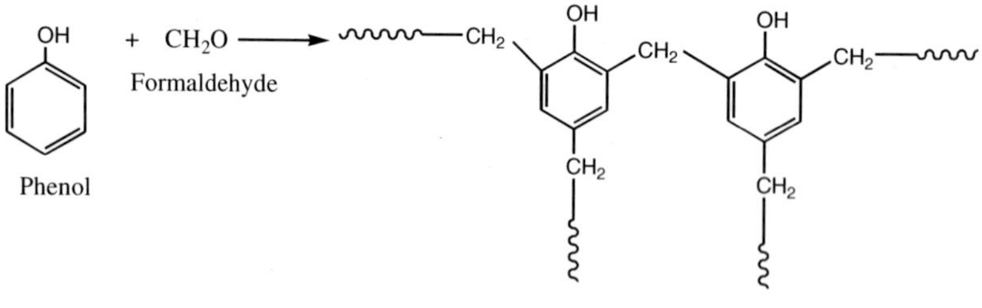

Figure 1.3. Reaction of Polycondensation of phenol and formaldehyde for the preparation of phenol - formaldehyde resins (Bakelite).

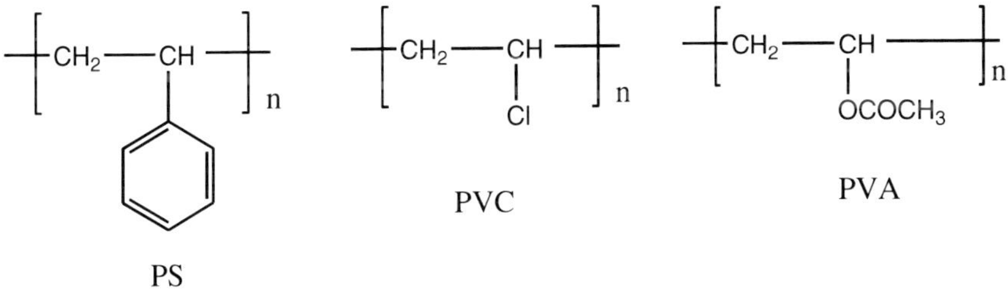

Figure 1.4. Chemical structure of polystyrene (PS), poly(vinyl chloride) (PVC) and poly(vinyl acetate) (PVA).

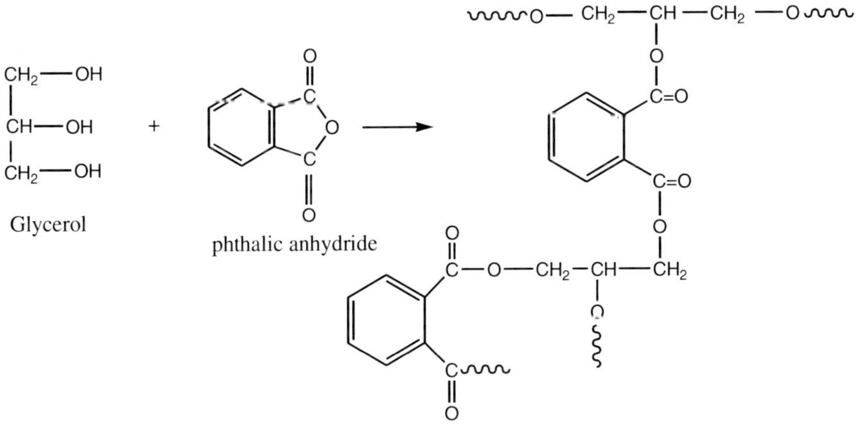

Figure 1.5. Reaction of polycondensation of glycerol with phthalic anhydride for preparation of an alkyd resin.

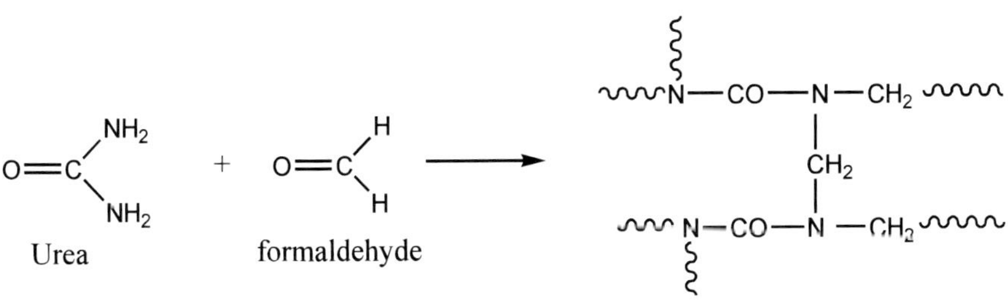

Figure 1.6. Reaction of polycondensation of urea with formaldehyde.

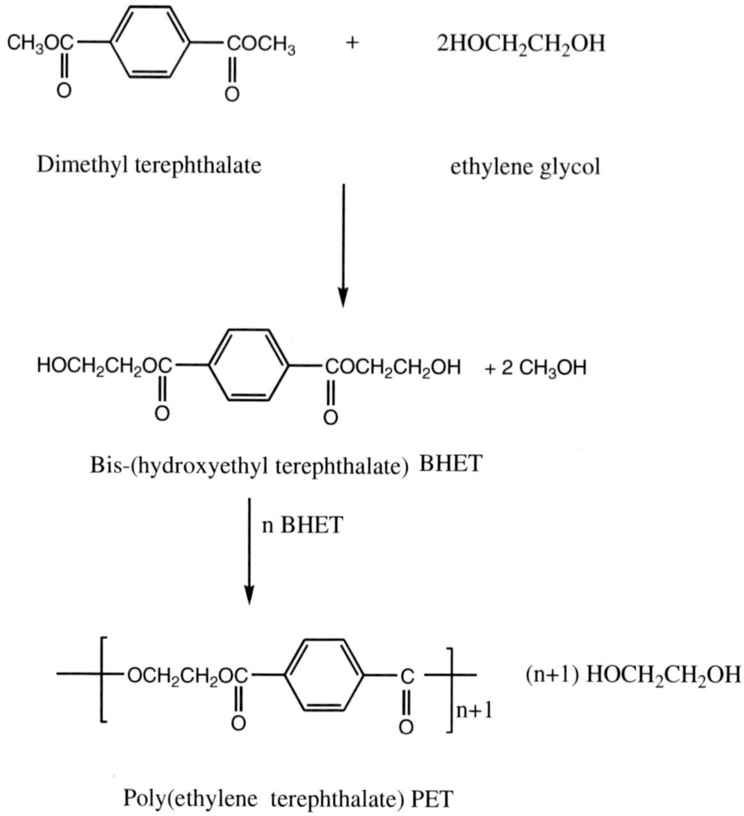

Figure 1.7. Polycondensation reactions for preparation of PET.

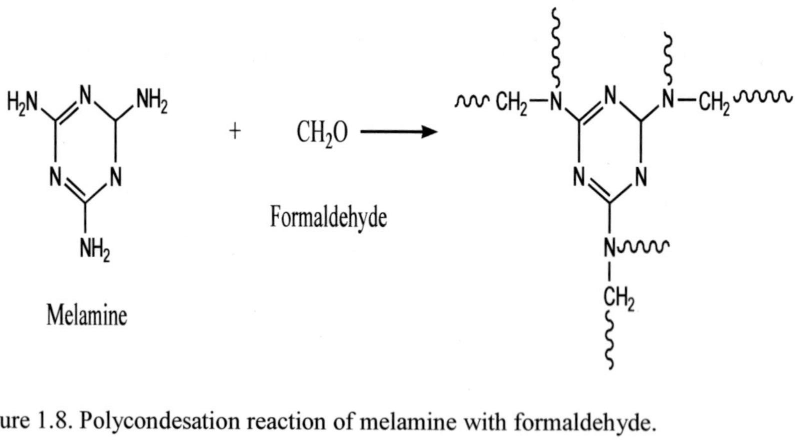

Figure 1.8. Polycondesation reaction of melamine with formaldehyde.

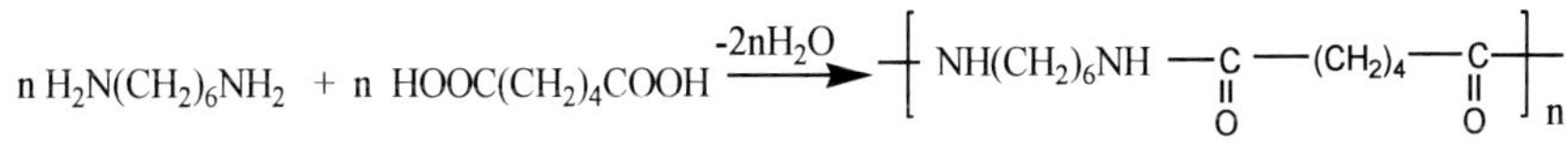

Figure 1.9. Polycondensation reaction of hexamethylene diamine and adipic acid for the preparation of Nylon 6,6 (1934).

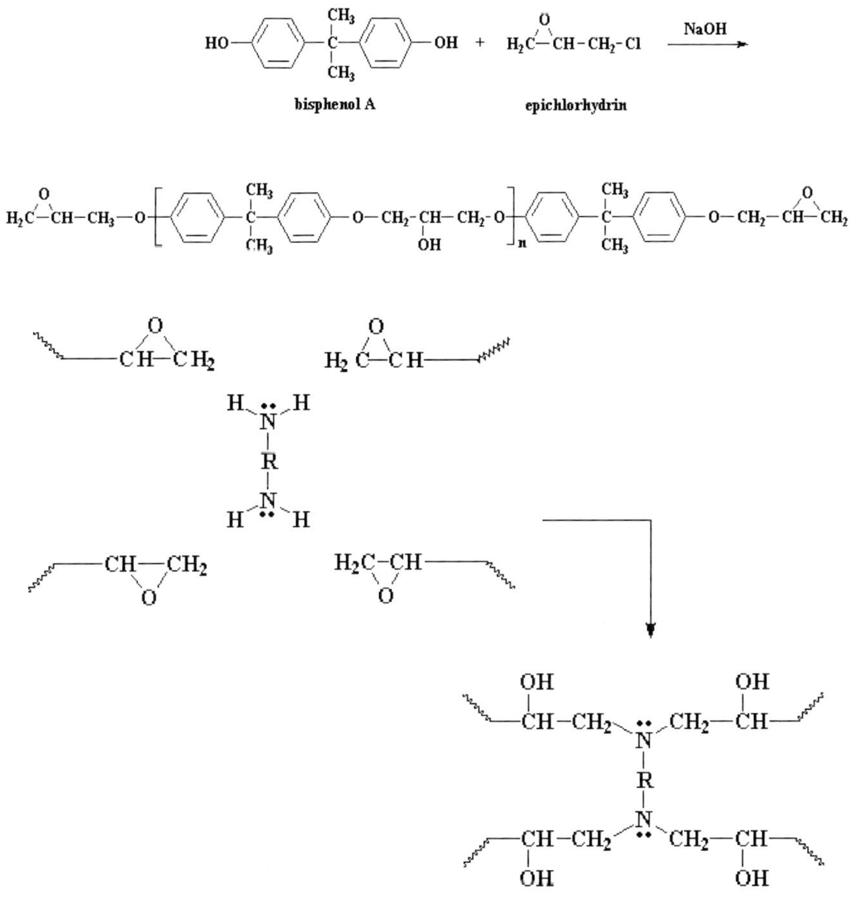

Figure 1.10. Reaction of bis-phenol A with epichlorydrine for the preparation of a diepoxide, which then reacts with a diamine to give a cross-linked epoxy resin.

Concurrent with the development of many of these synthetic materials was the proposal that they be used in dentistry. Much of the rapid development in polymer chemistry was driven by the desire to find a synthetic substitute for natural rubber, especially during World War I. The first, practical realization of this goal came in 1931 through the work of Wallace Carothers and others at Du Pont in the development of Neoprene. Neoprene is the trade name used by DuPont Performance Elastomers for the polymer prepared by polymerization of chloroprene (Figure 1.11). Neoprene or polychloroprene is an extremely versatile synthetic rubber with more than 75 years of proven performance in a broad industry spectrum. It was originally developed as an oil-resistant substitute for natural rubber. Neoprene is noted for a unique combination of properties, which has led to its use in thousands of applications in diverse environments.

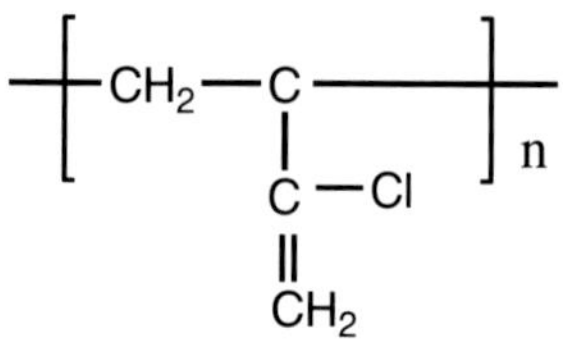

Figure 1.11. Chemical structure of Neoprene.

Of particular interest to the dental field is the development of acrylic chemistry. Acrylic acid (Figure 1.12) and its derivatives were well known, even by the 1890s. However, it was not until 1901, when Dr Otto Röhm, as a part of his PhD thesis, produced solid, transparent polymers of acrylic acid that this field started to emerge. Derivatives of acrylic monomers, methyl and ethyl acrylate (Figure 1.12), were made and also produced perfectly clear solid polymers. However, commercial development of these compounds was delayed because of a lack of a viable source for the monomers. By 1927, Acryloid (a non-yellowing substitute for nitrocellulose) and Plexigum (used in the early manufacture of safety glass), both polymers of poly(methyl acrylate) (Figure 1.13) were produced by Röhm and Haas as molding powders.

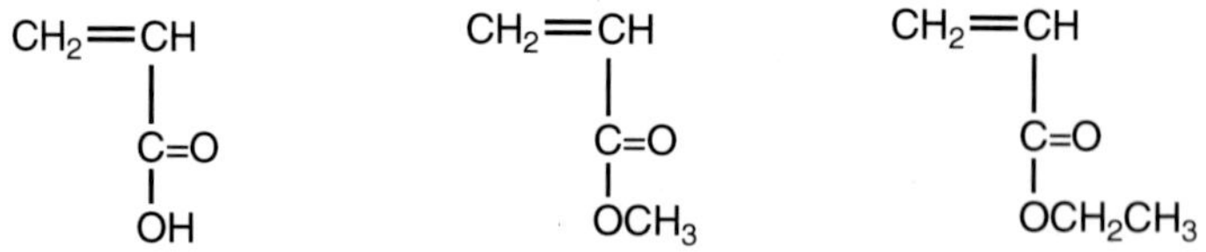

Acrylic Acid Methyl Acrylate Ethyl Acrylate

Figure 1.12. Chemical structure of acrylic acid and its methyl and ethyl ester.

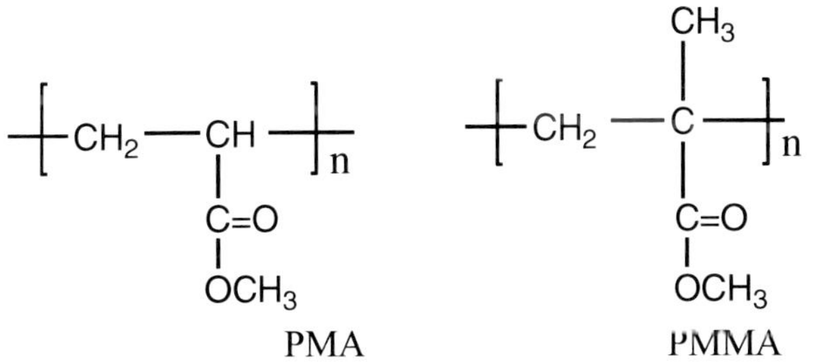

Figure 1.13. Chemical structure of poly(methyl acrylate) (PMA) and poly(methyl methacrylate) PMMA.

In 1931, commercial production of the harder poly(methyl methacrylate) (Figure 1.13) occurred, with introduction of Plexiglas (also known as organic glass, Lucite and Plexite) in sheet form. In 1932 Imperial Chemical Industries developed poly(methyl methacrylate) as a clearer and more durable form of safety glass (Perspex) in cast sheet form. By 1937, this material was also available in granules and molding powders. Du Pont and others utilized acrylic polymers in surface coatings, artificial leathers, fabric finishes, and acrylic-based paints; the latter essentially replaced oil-based paints for domestic use. Between 1930 and 1940, with the tremendous availability of a wide variety of easily attainable polymers, the dental profession used many polymers in the denture base field, only to find disappointment in the clinical arena. Many polymers were difficult to fabricate, in that they required expensive and complex laboratory equipment. The phenol-formaldehyde products were the first to compete with Vulcanite (Bakelite). These products were available in sheet, cake, and powder forms. However, the physical properties of the final denture base depended heavily on the processing techniques used. By 1932, mixtures of PVC and vinyl acetate were available for use as denture base materials, but the associated processing technique resulted in high residual stresses, and the base material often fractured shortly after case insertion.

The first practical replacement for Vulcanite as a denture base material came in 1936 with the introduction of Vernonite: a poly(methyl methacrylate) (PMMA) heat-processed material. Given the success of PMMA as a denture base, its use as a definitive restorative material was attempted as well. By 1940, Vernonite was being used for inlays, crowns, and fixed partial dentures. With the onset of World War II, further development in plastics continued, again with the goal of seeking a cheaper, synthetic alternative for the mass production of rubber. It has been estimated that by 1946, PMMA materials represented approximately 95% of the denture base market. It was not until after the war that room-temperature polymerization was made available and the so-called cold-, chemical-, or self-curing acrylics were used in dentistry. This change in polymerization method allowed, for the first time, the possibility of successfully placing a direct esthetic restorative material. Previous to this type setting reaction, practitioners attempted to place the powder and liquid components of the material directly into the cavity preparation. No chemical reaction resulted, only monomer penetration into the ground polymer powder, causing it to partially dissolve. Upon monomer evaporation, an intertwined mass of individual polymer chains remained, simulating a solid polymer mass. Room temperature polymerized materials relied upon an oxidation-reduction reaction (redox) in which, upon transfer of an electron among initiating agents, a free radical was formed at room temperature. Once this radical was formed, the polymerization process was started in a manner similar to that of the heat-polymerized materials. It was soon noticed that color stability of the polymerized restoration was a problem with self-curing systems. Research revealed that the color alteration arose from the use of amines as a co-initiator in the generation of free radicals. Enhanced color stability was achieved when the initiating system changed to a sulfinic acid reaction. However, even with improvement in color stability, it was found that these restorations did not hold up well clinically. The primary problems were related to volumetric shrinkage during polymerization within the preparation as well as the large difference in thermal expansion between the polymerized polymer and surrounding tooth structure. As a result of these difficulties, there was a high incidence of marginal staining and redecay along the restoration interface. The first tooth-colored, direct filling for anterior teeth using the sulfinic acid system appeared in the 1950s.

Attempts to enhance direct PMMA restorations did not completely resolve clinical issues. The biggest improvements in clinical performance of polymer based restorative materials came in the late 1950s and early 1960s. First, Dr Rafael Bowen started fundamental work on the use of high-molecular-weight epoxy and methacrylate-derivatives that incorporated inorganic filler loading. These materials were polymerized with the conventional redox methods of the cold-cure acrylic chemistry commonly used in restorative dentistry. The introduction of a high-molecular-weight, difunctional monomer (known as Bis-GMA or Bowen's resin) (Figure 1.14) greatly facilitated the commercial development of materials containing inorganic fillers: composites. The first uses of composite in paste/liquid form were developed by Robert Chang in 1969 and Henry Lee in 1970. Lee's development went on to commercialization and was known as *Adaptic* (Johnson and Johnson, New

Brunswick, N.J.) a paste/paste material. It should be noted that the monomeric content of these systems did not rely completely on the use of Bis-GMA. This monomer is extremely viscous due to the presence of two hydroxyl groups that provide significant intermolecular hydrogen bonding. To solve this viscosity issue, manufacturers typically diluted the monomer with a more fluid co-monomer, the triethylene glycol dimethacrylate (TEGDMA) (Figure 1.14). In 1965 Bowen patented the combination of Bis-GMA resin and silane-treated quartz particles, which is the origin of most polymer composites on the market today. These polymer composites have been the subject of considerable academic research and are now used widely in operative dentistry. Polymer composites together with glass-ionomer cements (invented in 1969 and first clinically tested in the early 1970s) have a wider application than any other restorative material available to the dental profession.

The introduction of photo-polymerization of dental resins in the mid-1970s started a new era in operative dentistry. At the end of the 1970s the first UV-light cured resin, Novalight (L.D. Caulk) was introduced on the market.

Hence the last 50 years has seen the proliferation of both the number and chemical sophistication of polymeric dental materials. This has involved the study of a wide range of material properties, some of which are common with materials as a whole and others specific to dentistry. The continuing growth of regulatory requirements with respect to toxicity adds an extra dimension to the development of dental materials.

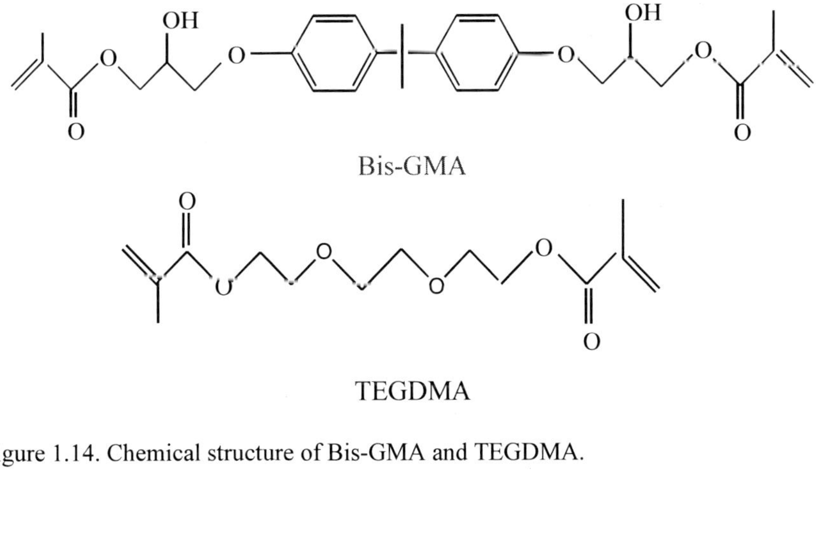

Figure 1.14. Chemical structure of Bis-GMA and TEGDMA.

1.1. LITERATURE

[1] Bascones, A.; Vega, J.M.; Olmo, N.; Turnay, J.; Gavilanes, J.G.; Lizarbe, M.A. Dental and Maxillofacial Surgery Applications of Polymers. In Editor, Severian Dumitriu. *Polymeric Biomaterials (Second Edition, Revised and Expanded)*. New York: Marcel Dekker; 2001; 423-450.

[2] Rueggeberg, F.A. 2002. From vulcanite to vinyl, a history of resins in restorative dentistry. *J Prosthet Dent* , 87, 364-79.

Chapter 2

POLYMERIC DENTAL PROSTHETIC MATERIALS

2.1. DENTURE BASES

A denture consists of artificial teeth set in a denture base which retains the artificial teeth and rests on the soft tissues of the mouth. The first non metallic denture base material which was used with some success was vulcanite (vulcanized rubber) supplied in the form of a plastic sheet impregnated with some 32% sulfur. This sheet was cut up and packed in the mould space and polymerized under heat (168 °C) and pressure (620 kN/m^2). This material lasted in popularity for some 80 or more years and was displaced as the front runner in this field by (PMMA) which was introduced in the 1930s. With vulcanite the aesthetics were poor due to the opacity allow bacterial proliferation and dimensional changes occurred during polymerization, about 4% contraction. Other synthetic polymers which were used for denture bases are Bakelite (phenol-formaldehyde) cellulose nitrate, nylon, epoxy resins and vinyl polymers such as poly(vinyl chloride), poly(vinyl acetate) and polystyrene. Polycarbonates containing up to glass fibers of 150 μm length and 10 μm diameter have been used for denture construction. These polymers have remarkably good impact properties, up to nine times better than poly(methyl methacrylate). These materials are more difficult to mold dentally than acrylics, since injection molding is required.

Ideally a denture base material should possess the following properties [1]:

1. *Biological properties.* It should be non-toxic and non-irritant, chemically inert or at least compatible with the oral tissues.
2. *Chemical properties.* It should be unaffected by oral fluids, that is, it should be insoluble, non-absorbent and inert. It should not have a taste or odor and should not pick up a taste or odor from oral fluids.
3. *Mechanical properties.* It should have adequate mechanical properties, for example:
    - High modulus of elasticity, so that greater rigidity can be achieved, even in comparatively thin sections of material.
    - High proportional limit, so that the denture will not easily undergo permanent deformation when stressed.
    - High strength, this is frequently measured as the transverse strength.
    - Have resilience strength sufficient to permit the use of a thin base.
    - High impact strength, so that the denture will not fracture if accidentally dropped, or fracture if the wearer is involved in an accident.
    - High fatigue strength.
    - Hard and with good abrasion resistance, so that the material will not wear appreciably, but will take and retain a high polish.
4. *Other physical properties.*
    - The thermal expansion of the denture base should match that of the tooth material.
    - The thermal conductivity should be high.
    - The density should be low to assist in the retention of an upper denture.
    - The softening temperature should be higher than the temperature of liquids and foods in the mouth.
5. *Esthetic properties.* As a matter of prime importance, the material should be esthetically satisfactory. The material should be transparent or translucent and easily pigmented. Be capable of being colored to match the various mucosa colors and retain this color with time, use and cleansing.
6. *Other properties.*
    - Radiopacity. A denture base material must have radiopacity. If a denture or a fragment of a broken denture is accidentally inhaled or ingested, it should be capable of detection on radiographs.

- A denture base material should be easy to process with the minimum of expense and equipment.
- It should be easy to repair if accidentally fractured; it be capable of being repaired and relined/rebased by customary dental techniques.
- There should be no dimensional changes (expansion, contraction or warpage) either on processing the denture or while it is in service.
- Be capable of being cleaned by usual oral hygiene techniques and materials. Not soften or wrap in hot water or other cleansing solutions.

There is no denture base material which meets all of these requirements. However, the currently used denture base materials are very satisfactory. Dentures are constructed individually for each person to the requirements defined by an appropriate impression of the mouth and the various dimensions recorded. The geometry and size of each denture will vary. Each denture base will lie against tissue-some hard (such as the enamel of a tooth) and some soft (such as the mucosa and soft tissues that cover the bone of the jaws). In addition, each denture is subject to loading in both chewing and non-chewing contacts.

A complete denture is entirely supported by soft tissues and when loaded will flex in a complex manner that is partially determined by the uneven thickness of the mucosal base. It is difficult to estimate the number of flexures that a denture might undergo, but it is possible to suggest that a denture might flex about one million times per year. The amount of flexure will be limited by the compressibility of the mucosa and could be up to about 1 mm across the posterior dimension of a complete upper denture. Due to the low fracture strength of poly(methyl methacrylate) these dentures may fracture easily in use in high strain rate situations. It has been proposed that poly(methyl methacrylate) dentures made for the upper jaw are liable to fracture in a fatigue mode, but the evidence is not entirely conclusive. It is possible, however that the bone of the jaws will resorb and if this should happen in the upper jaw then flexure could be great. In the upper jaw, bone loss will occur on the ridges, that is, on the outer aspect, but not centrally in the palate. The denture will then flex about its center line more when the resorption is greater. This is the clinical situation that could lead to clinical fatigue failure, particularly when a centrally placed incisal notch is present at the front of the denture [2].

2.1.1. Physical Form and Composition

Denture base materials commonly are supplied as a powder to be mixed with a liquid, which is then molded under heat and pressure to form dentures. Most commercial materials contain *poly(methyl methacrylate)* usually as beads, manufactured by emulsion polymerization of methyl methacrylate, 35-200 μm in diameter. Small proportions of ethyl, butyl or other alkyl methacrylates may copolymerize with methyl methacrylate to create a more fracture resistant product. Other manufactures may add small quantities (<5%) of ethyl acrylate to increase solubility and to improve flow properties in the molten state. The powder also contains *benzoyl peroxide* (0.5 to 1.5%) to initiate the polymerization of the monomer liquid after being added to the powder. *A cross-linking agent,* such as ethylene glycol dimethacrylate, is essential to improve hardness and wear resistance of the final product.

Pure polymers, such as poly(methyl methacrylate) are clear and are adaptable to a wide range of pigmentation. The pigments used to obtain the various tissue-like shades are compounds such as mercuric sulfide, cadmium sulfide, cadmium selenide, ferric oxide or carbon black, although the use of cadmium salts is suspect because of demonstrated toxicity. These pigments may be locked into the polymer beads by addition during the commercial polymerization, or they may be mechanically mixed with the polymer beads after polymerization. Generally, the latter method is used and the uneven distribution of the pigment in the final denture gives a mottled, natural-appearing denture. Dyes, as well pigments, occasionally are used, but generally they are not as satisfactory, because they tend to leach out of the plastic by the oral fluids, which results in a gradual lightening of the shade. In addition to coloring agents, zinc or titanium oxides are used as opacifiers, with titanium dioxide being the most effective. Dyed synthetic fibers made from nylon or acrylic usually are added to the denture material to simulate the minute blood vessels underlying the oral mucosa [2].

2.2. Denture Relines

After a new denture has been inserted, it ought to retain in the mouth quite nicely due to the fact that the shape of the inside of the denture base conforms closely to the shape of the gums. Unfortunately, the longer you wear the denture, the more your gums change underneath it, and the looser it gets. In order to restore the retentive qualities of the denture, and to prevent the production of flabby gum tissue under it, you should have the denture professionally relined at least every two years. There are actually three types of denture relines: Hard, Soft and Temporary.

2.2.1. Hard Relines

This is the kind of reline that should be done on all full dentures every two years. The dentist removes some of the plastic from the inside of the denture, and then fills the denture with a soft material (think of soft putty) which, when replaced in the mouth, conforms to the contours of the tissues, and then hardens to a rubbery consistency. When the denture is removed, the denture now contains an accurate impression of the shape of the gums. The denture is sent to the lab, and the impression material is replaced with pink, hard acrylic in exactly the same shape as the original impression material. When returned, the denture now conforms to the contours of your mouth and should make maximum contact with the tissues producing maximum suction. In our office, the impression is scheduled for first thing in the morning. The patient goes home without the denture, but returns later the same day (usually early afternoon) for the insert (fitting appointment) [3]

The reline can be achieved either with a cold-cure acrylic resin at the chairside, or the denture is sent to a dental laboratory for relining with a heat-cured acrylic. The heat-cured acrylics used by laboratories are identical to those used for the construction of dentures. The cold-cured come in two types with constituents as listed in Table 2.1. The reason for the second type of reline material is that MMA is very iritant to soft tissues and can sensitize the patient. Poly (ethyl methacrylate) (PEMA) and butyl methacrylate are less irritant to the patient, but have the disadvantage that they cause a reduction in the T_g , and this increases the possibility of dimensional instability [4].

One of the most serious drawbacks to attempting a chairside reline is that there is little control over the amount of denture material removed and the thickness of the reline material that replaces it. Other problems include high exothermic reactions, unacceptable taste and poor colour stability over time [4].

Table 2.1. The two types of cold-cured resin [4]

	Type I	Type II
Powder	Poly(methyl methacrylate) Benzoyl peroxide Pigments	Poly(ethyl methacrylate) Benzoyl peroxide Pigments
Liquid	Methyl methacrylate Di-n-butylphthalate Amine	Butyl methacrylate Amine

2.2.2. Soft Relines

In our rapidly aging society, the number of patients with difficulties in complete denture treatment, including highly absorbed alveolar ridges, is increasing. In the case of an extremely resorbed residual ridge, the overlying mucosa decreases in thickness according to the resorption. As the shock absorbing effect of the mucosa is diminished and masticatory impact forces are directly transmitted to the underlying tissue, the burden on the residual ridge is increased. In addition lesions, generalized irritation, or soreness are seen on the basal seat, because the thin mucosa is pinched between the hard denture base and the bone during mastication. In such caes, it is necessary to line the inner surface of the denture base with a soft material similar to the mucosa in order to compensate for the lost thickness and viscoelasticity of the mucosa. The pain is relieved by reducing the impact force during mastication and disprsing the force widely over the alveolar ridge to give a cush ioning effect. The application of a soft lining material to the mandibular denture can also increase the patient's masticatory performance and biting force and moreover improve the chewing rhythm [5].

Polymers with a glass transition temperature just above the temperature in the mouth will have a rubbery behavior and are highly resilient. Some polymers have a naturally low glass transition temperature (e.g. silicon polymers) and others (e.g. PMMA) can be modified by the inclusion of plasticizers to reduce their glass transition temperature. The plasticizer acts as a lubricant for the polymer chains, making it easier for them to slide past one another, allowing the material to deform more easily and giving it a lower elastic modulus.

The ideal properties of a soft lining material include the following [6]:

1. Biocompatibility –non-toxic and non-irritant to the oral tissues.
2. Permanently compliant-soft enough for the comfort of the patient.
3. Permanently resilient-the actual level of resilience required is unknown as shown by the range available.
4. Adhere to the denture base and remain so in the mounth.
5. Low water uptake-a high uptake will cause distortion and may result in fouling of the lining due to ingress of bacteria etc.; similar level to that of the denture base is ideal ~2-3%.
6. Wetted by saliva-a thin film of saliva is necessary for the retention of the denture and to act as a lubricant to prevent irritation of the mucosa.
7. Should not support the growth of *Candida albicans* –this is a common yeast responsible for causing denture stomatitis, a common occurrence in denture wearers.
8. Sufficient mechanical properties-enough to withstand normal handling, brushing etc.
9. Easy to clean-not adversely be affected by denture cleansers, not stained easily etc.

The majority of soft lining materials currently available can be classified into two main types, soft acrylic and silicon rubber.

Acrylic Soft Lining Materials

These soft liners have the advantage that they adhere strongly to the PMMA denture. They can be subdivided into those containing leachable plasticizers and those containing polymerizable plasticizers.

Leachable Plasticizer Systems

Poly(ethyl methacrylate) (PEMA) has a T_g of only 66°C, compared with 100 °C for PMMA. A combination of these two polymers, wth a small amount of plasticizer, such as dibutylphthalate, is highly resilient. Thus the powder is a mixture of PEMA and PMMA and the liquid is MMA, containing 25-50% plasticizer. Unfortunately, the plasticizer gradually leaches out and the liner becomes stiff as it loses its resilience. How rapidly this transition takes place depends to some extent on the patient's regime for cleaning the denture. In general, high temperatures and strong bleaching agents shoud be avoided [4]

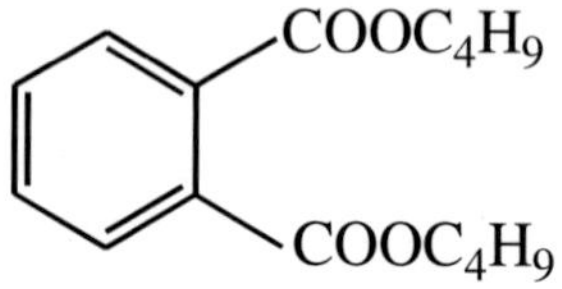

Dibutyl phthalate

Polymerizable Plasticizer Systems

New plasticizers have been developed that polymerise and thus resist dissolution, but which maintain their lubricating effect. Exact formulations of this new material are not known, but some use alkyl maleate or alkyl itaconate, while for one experimental system the liquid component is known to be a mixture of tridecyl methacrylate, 2-diethylhexyl maleate and ethylene glycol dimethacrylate. The liquid is mixed with either PEMA or copolymers of n-butyl and ethyl methacrylate. The material is fairy hard at room temperature, which makes it easy to finish and softens when taken up to mouth temperature [4].

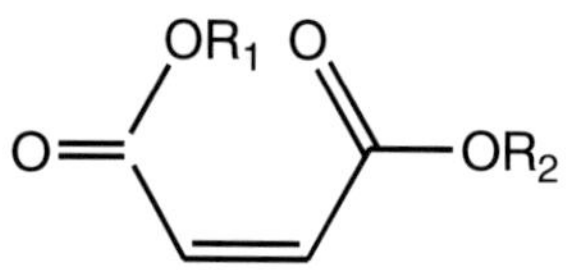

Alkyl maleate

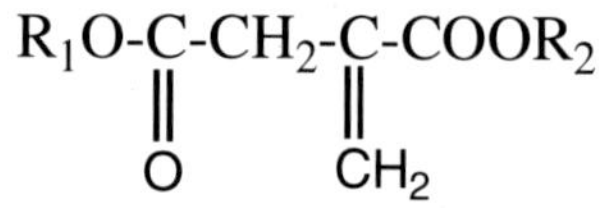

alkyl itaconate

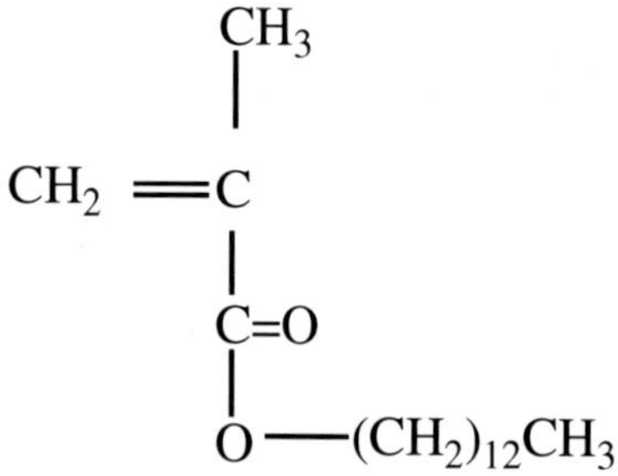

Tridecyl methacrylate

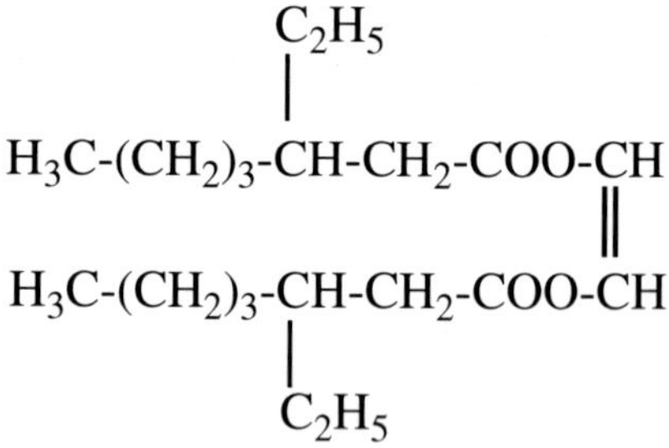

Di-2-2-ethylhexyl maleate

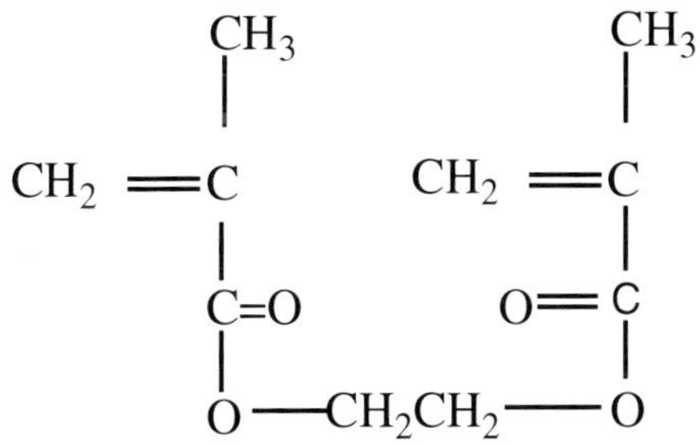

Ethylene glycol dimethacrylate

Silicon Soft Lining Materials

The silicon rubber consists of a poly(dimethyl siloxane) to which filler is added to give it the correct consistency. The material solidifies by a crosslinking process which can be achieved at room temperature with the use of a crosslinking agent or by heat

Room Temperature Polymerizing Materials

This type is basically a two-past system based on a hydroxyl-terminated poly(dimethyl siloxane) with an alkoxy orthosilicate cross-linking agent and organo-tin catalyst. The main problem with this type of material is lack of bonding to the PMMA denture base and as such they are usually supplied with and adhesive. This comprises a silicon polymer in a solvent, but even with its use the degree of bonding is still less than that of the soft acrylic materials. They also have a number of other drawbacks, such as supporting the growth of *Candida albicans* and having a large water uptake. One such material Flexibase (Flexico Developments Ltd., England) was found to have an uptake of ~50 wt%! This is somewhat surprisingas silicon polymers are hydrophobic. However, transport of water through them is rapid and the high uptake is due to a combination of this and the presence of hydrophilic filler particles commonly used in silico rubber materials [6].

Heat Polymerizing System

One material crosslinked with heat is the Molloplast B (Karl Huber GmbH&Co. KG, Germany).It is a one-paste system which consists of an acetoxy-cure silicon material (RTV 108) (720 parts), PMMA (19.15 parts), γmethacryloxypropyltrimethoxysilane (A 174) (9.16 parts) and titanium dioxide and washung red (0.075 parts) [7]. Obviously the past has to be mixed under dry conditions to prevent the RTV 108 polymerizing. During the mixing there must be a reaction to produce a stable paste. It is suggested that the acetoxy-Si groups from the RTV 108 react with the methoxy-Si groups from the silane A174. However, the situation is a little more complex as the A174 is only added as a minor component (~1.22%) and it also has a role in cross-linking and bonding to the denture base. Molloplast B, unlike the room temperature polymerizing silicones, does adhere to the denture by way of the methacrylate group on the silane A174. This has been improved by use of an adhesive, probably just the silane A174. Molloplast B also has low water uptake, however it does have low tear energy, which is a common problem with silicon rubbers.

Elastomer/Methacrylate Systems

A combination of an elastomer with a methacrylate monomer is commercially available with the trade name Novus (Hygenic Corp) which shows good strength and adhesion to the PMMA denture. It is a one-paste system containing a poly(fluoralkoxy)phosphazine elastomer: (PNF 200, Firestone) [8].

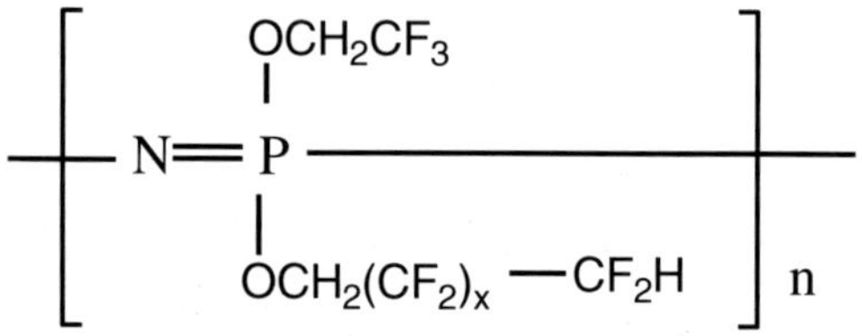

PNF 200

The paste is producing by milling the elastomer with the methacrylate monomers (trimethylolpropanentrimethacrylate, ethylene glycol dimethacrylate) acting as crosslinking agents, PMMA acting as filler, BaSO4 (radiopaque filler), lauroyl peroxide acting as initiator, and CdSSE dark red (pigment). As crosslinking will occur, albeit very slowly even at low temperatures the paste needs refrigerating or even freezing. The paste is rather stiff and does require careful moulding and its elastic nature requires the uncured material to be left in the mould to relax prior to heat curing.

2.2.3. Temporary Relines/Tissue Conditioners

Frequently, by the time a patient with an old denture finally shows up at the dentist's office looking for a new denture, the dentures have not been serviced for such a long time that the gums are in terrible condition. They may be red, swollen and quite misshapen. Relining the old denture, or building a new one using impressions taken while the gums are in such poor condition would lead to a denture that would simply perpetuate the problem with the new appliance.

When faced with situations like this, a dentist will frequently resort to a temporary, or palliative (medicated) reline material to allow the inflammation to subside. This reline makes the denture fit much more tightly, and is usually soft and pliable. It will not last more than a few months, but the patient wears it for a few weeks until the gums return to a more normal state. After this happens, then the patient is ready for the new denture or *hard reline* [3].

A temporary lining may be used for one of two purposes. Firstly, it may be a *tissue conditioner*; this may be define as a soft material that is applied temporarily to the fitting surface of a denture in order to allow a more equal distribution of load, to permit the mucosal tissues to assume a more normal position. Secondly, temporary lining materials may be used as *functional impression materials*. These are applied to the fitting surface of dentures in order to secure impressions under functional stresses.

Tissue conditioners and functional impression materials should have no irritant or toxic effect. The set materials for each of the two applications being considered have different requirements [1]:

Table 2.2. Components of a typical tissue conditioner

Powder	Liquid
Poly(ethyl methacrylate) or	Aromatic ester, usually a phthalate e.g
Copolymer of ethyl methacrylate with methyl or butyl methacrylate	butyl phthalyl butyl glycolate or dibutyl phthalate.
	Others used include benzyl benzoate and benzyl salicate + 6-30% ethanol

1. A tissue conditioner must be soft and it must not undergo substantial permanent deformation that is it must be elastic. The softness and elasticity must be maintained for a sufficient length of time.
2. A functional impression material should also be soft but must deform plastically to record the impression.

Many of the materials used for these two applications are viscoelastic that is, they flow under steady pressure, but are resilient under dynamic forces such as chewing.

They are generally presented as a powder and liquid system composition as shown in Table 2.2. When the powder and liquid are mixed the ethanol swells the polymer beads and allows penetration by the ester plasticizer. As a result a gel is formed by polymer chain entanglement [9]. The resulting gel is viscoelastic in that it responds elastically to the rapid dynamic loading associated with masticationbut will flow under constant fluid loads [10]. In fact it acts like a Maxwell fluid.

In the mouth first the ethanol and then the plasticizer is lost, resulting in hardening of the material [11],[12]. It is necessary that, when used as a tissue conditioner, it should be replaced every 2-3 days. However as a temporary reline material it can be used for up to 3 months, depending on the material. As a functional impression material it is recommended that it be in place for at least 24h [13]. Bonding to the denture is good which makes them difficult to remove, a problem if regular replacement is required.

The leached ethanol can cause further irritation of traumatized tissues, especially in the high ethanol content materials. Leached plasticizer is a cause for concern over possible toxicity as with the soft acrylic, especially as the plasticizer content is higher. The leached plasticizer can also cause problems by plasticizing adjacent denture base materials. This will reduce rigidity and make the denture more prone to fracture [6].

2.3. CROWN AND BRIDGE MATERIALS

These materials are used as interim tooth coverage during fabrication of permanent prostheses. They should maintain the correct biting relationship, stop teeth drifting and protect the prepared tooth against pulpal irritation and fracture. The materials are based on methyl methacrylate, higher methacrylates (ethyl, or isobutyl) and “epimine” polymers [14].

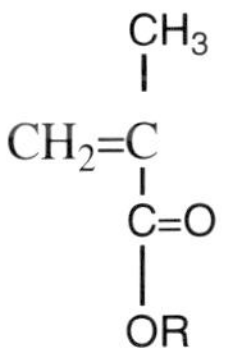

R= CH_3 (methyl methacrylate, MMA)

R= CH_2CH_3 (ethyl methacrylate, EMA

R= CH_2CHCH_3 (isobutyl methacrylate, i-BuMA)
CH_3

Materials based on poly(methyl methacrylate) have the advantage of the low cost, good wear resistance, good esthetics, high polishability,and good color stability. However they have the disadvantage of significant amount of heat given off by exothermic polymerization reaction of MMA, high degree of shrinkage (about 8%), strong objectionable odor, short working time, hard to repair, must be mixed, radiolucent. Materials based on poly (ethyl- or isobutyl methacrylate) have the advantage of low cost, less heat given off during polymerization reaction than poly(methyl methacrylate), less shrinkage than poly(methyl methacrylate), and extended working time. They have the disadvantages: less esthetic than other currently-marketed materials, poor wear resistance, poor color stability, strong, objectionable odor, hard to repair, must be mixed, radiolucent.

Epimine was ccommercially introduced in 1968 as a two-component paste composed of a difunctional ethyleneimine-termined high molecular weight monomer with filler and a liquid containing a benzene sulfonate cationic initiator [15].

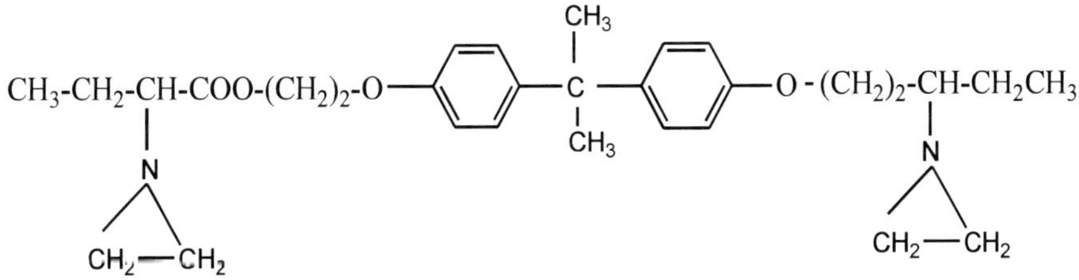

The imine ring is opened by R+ ions from the liquid ininiator of cationic polymerization:

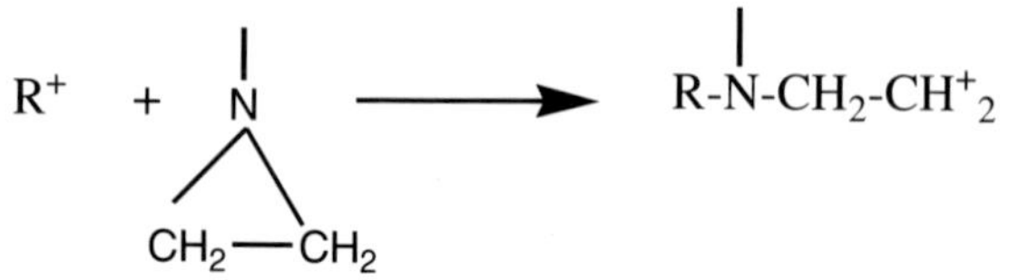

Epimine resins are not as strong as methacrylate resins, but exhibit good flow, low exotherm and low curing shrinkage.

2.4. Polymer Cements

Dental cements are hard, brittle materials formed by mixing powder and liquid together. Dental cements are used for a variety of dental and orthodontic applications, including use as luting agents, pulp-protecting agents or cavity-lining material. Furthermore, they are used to form an insulating layer under metallic or ceramic restorations, and protect the pulp from injury. This helps in sealing or fixing and casting inlays, onlays or any such substance to both dentin and enamel.

Cements are classified on the basis of their components. Generally, they can be classified into categories:

- Metals (amalgam): mercury and, generally, silver
- Water-based: zinc phosphate ($Zn_3(PO_4)_2$),
- Zinc Polyacrylate (or Zinc Polycarboxylate), glass ionomer cement (GIC)
- Oil-based: Zinc oxide eugenol and Non-eugenol zinc oxide.

Zinc oxide eugenol (ZOE) is a material created by the combination of zinc oxide and eugenol. Eugenol ($C_{10}H_{12}O_2$), is an allyl chain-substituted guaiacol. Eugenol is a member of the phenylpropanoids class of chemical compounds. It is a clear to pale yellow oily liquid extracted from certain essential oils especially from clove oil, nutmeg, cinnamon, and bay leaf. It is slightly soluble in water and soluble in organic solvents. It has a pleasant, spicy, clove-like aroma.

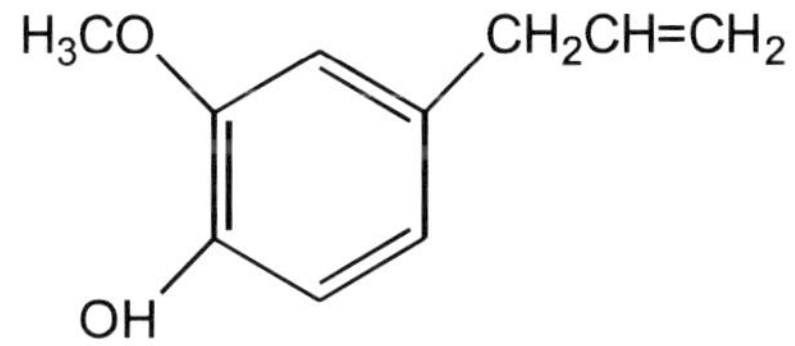

Eugenol

Zinc oxide eugenol (ZOE) is a material created by the combination of zinc oxide and eugenol (contained in oil of cloves) which can be used as a filling or cement material in dentistry.[1][2] It is often used in dentistry when the decay is very deep or very close to the nerve or pulp chamber. Because the tissue inside the tooth, i. e. the pulp, reacts badly to the drilling stimulus (heat and vibration), it frequently becomes severely inflamed and precipitates a condition called acute or chronic pulpitis. This condition usually leads to severe chronic tooth sensitivity or actual toothache and can then only be treated with the removal of the nerve (pulp) called root canal therapy. The placement of a ZOE "temporary" for a few to several days prior to the placement of the final filling usually prevents the sensitivity or toothache and therefore, most times, precludes the need for the expensive and time consuming root canal procedure. It is classified as an intermediate restorative material and has anaesthetic and antibacterial properties. It is sometimes used in the management of dental caries as a "temporary filling". ZOE cements were introduced in the 1980s.

- Resin-based: acrylate or methacrylate resin cements, including the latest generation of self-adhesive resin cements which contain silicate or other types of fillers in an organic resin matrix.

Cements can be classified based on the type of their matrix:

- Phosphate (zinc phosphate, silicon phosphate)
- Zinc Polyacrylate (or Zinc Polycarboxylate), glass ionomer cement (GIC)
- Phenolate (Zinc oxide–eugenol and 2-Ethoxybenzoic acid)
- Resin (polymeric)

Another classification takes into account the main component; those containing zinc oxide powder include zinc oxide, zinc phosphate and zinc silicophosphate cements. Cements containing leachable glass powder are GIC, silicate and silicophosphate. Less commonly used cements include those containing liquid polyacrylic acid (resin cement) and those containing phosphoric acid (zinc phosphate cement).

The requirements for dental cements are that they should:

- Be non irritant to pulp and gingiva (gums) and should not support the growth of secondary caries. (This last property is called cariostatic or anticariogenicity).
- Form a strong bond with enamel and dentin.
- Provide good marginal sealing to prevent marginal leakage.
- Be resistant to dissolution in saliva, or in any other oral fluid.
- Have good aesthetics and good thermal and chemical resistance. (Opacity to X-rays is also preferred for diagnostic purposes). [16].

2.4.1. Zinc Polyacrylate (Polycarboxylate) Cements

The zinc polyacrylate cements also referred to as zinc polycarboxylate are supplied as a powder and a liquid or as a powder that is mixed with water. The liquid is a water solution of poly(acrylic acid) which has the following chemical structure:

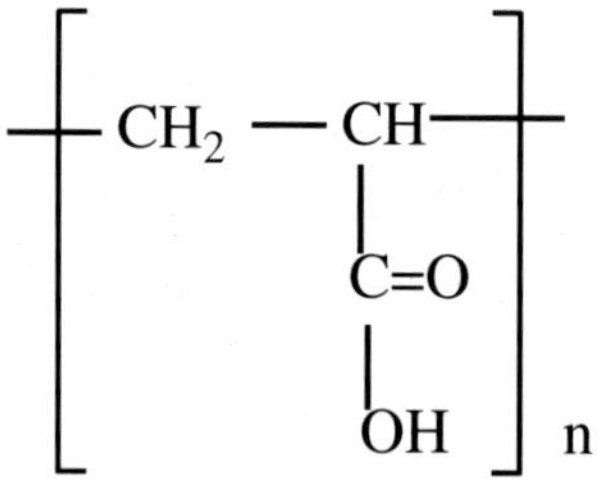

Most commercial liquids are supplied as a 32% 42% solution of poly(acrylic acid) having a molecular weight of 25,000 to 50,000. The manufacturer control the viscosity of the cement liquid by varying the molecular weight of the polymer or by adjusting the pH by adding sodiul hydroxide. Itaconic acid and tartaric acid may be present to stabilize the liquid, which can gel on extended storage.

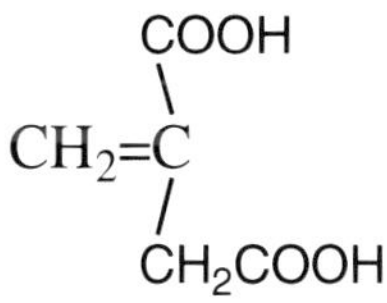

Itaconic acid

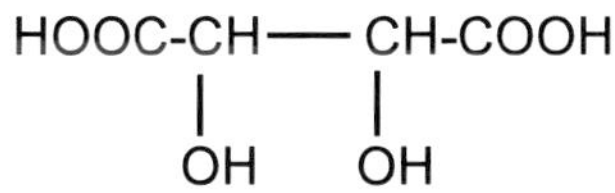

Tartaric acid

The cement powder is essentially zinc oxide and magnesium oxide that have been sintered and ground to reduce the reactivity of zinc oxide. The cement powder that is mixed with water contains 15% to 18% poly(acrylic acid) coated on the oxide particles [2]. The structure of the set cement has been studied in detail. Early indications, using infrared spectroscopy, were that this material was purely ionic, with Zn^{2+} ions showing no interaction with the adjacent carboxylate groups [17]. However this proved to be an artifact of the poor resolution of technique, because when this material was studied using FTIR a complex array of structural types were detected, all showing some partial covalency in the interaction of Zn^{2+} ions with carboxylate groups [18]

The various structures proposed are illustrated in Figure 2.1. [19]

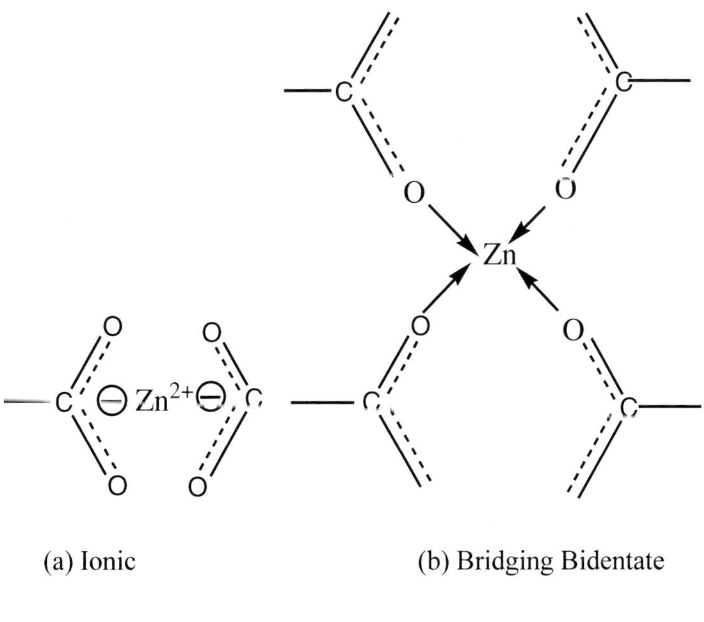

(a) Ionic (b) Bridging Bidentate

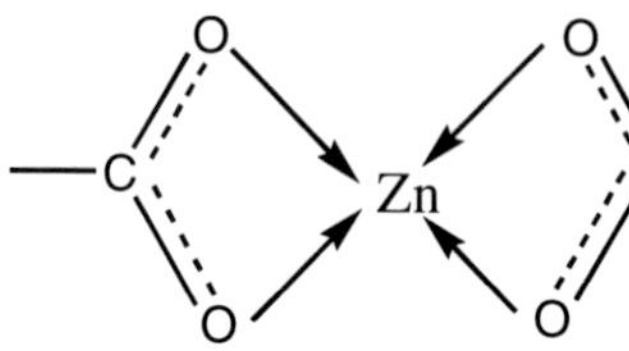

(c) Chelating Bidentate

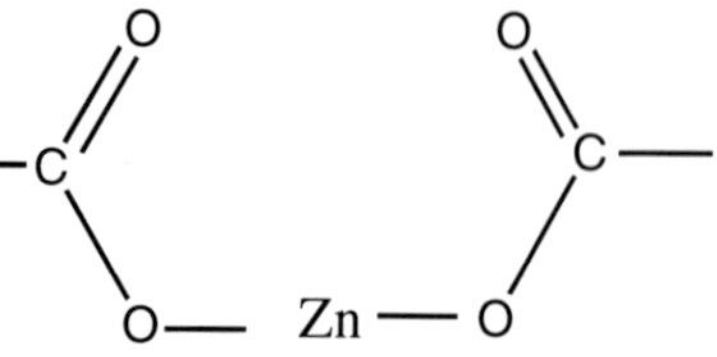

(d) Asymmetric unidentate

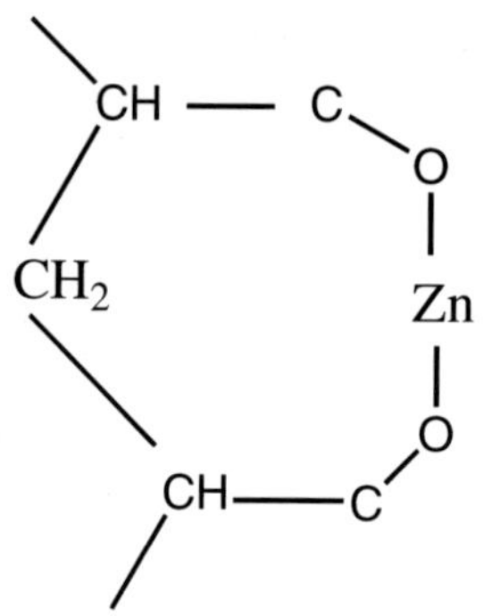

(e) Chelate bidentate (8-membered ring)

Figure 2.1. Possible chelate structures occurring in zinc polycarboxylate dental cements [19].

The role of water in these materials has been studied in some detail. Water is involved in the setting reaction, because it is needed to dissolve the poly(acrylic acid). Since setting takes place withpout phase separation, it is known that water remains within the set cement, at least under normal circumstances. Storing these cements under desiccating conditions, either dry air [20] or in saturated salt solutions [21] causes these cements to lose considerable amounts of mass, presumably due to loss of water, but this has not been found to affect their compressive strength. This led to the conclusion that water, which probably occupies co-ordination sites around the around the zinc ions and the polyanions, does not have a structural role [19].

An important property of zinc polyacrylate cements is their adhesion to dentine and enamel, which enables them to be used as dental adhesives. Zinc polyacrylate cements are used primarily for luting permanent restorations and as bases. These cements have also been used in orthodontics for cementation of bands and at one time for direct bonding of brackets and in endodontics as a root canal filling material [19].

2.4.2. Glass-ionomer Cements (GICs)

"Glass- ionomer cements" (or more correctly "glass-polyalkenoate") are materials made of calcium, strontium aluminosilicate glass powder (base) combined with a water soluble polymer (acid). When the components are mixed together, they undergo a setting reaction involving neutralization of the acid groups by the powdered solid glass base. Because both components are materials of wide chemical diversity, the range of glass-ionomer cements is very wide indeed and the material has considerable potential for further development. There are a number of applications for these cements and accordingly they are classified:

Type I:	Luting crowns, bridges and orthodontic brackets
Type II a:	Aesthetic restorative cements
Type II b:	Reinforced restorative cements
Type III:	Lining cements, Base

The chemistry is essentially the same for all three categories and involves a significant acid-base reaction as a part of setting reaction and show a continuing fluoride release; but there are variations in powder/liquid ratio and powder particle size to accommodate the desired function [22].

Glass- ionomer cements have certain advantages, such as they bond adhesively to enamel and dentin, release fluoride ions over a prolonged period of time, are biocompatible and have approximately the same coefficient of thermal expansion as that of tooth structure. However, in spite of these advantages conventional glass-ionomer cements suffer from the disadvantages such as short working time and rather long setting time, brittleness, low fracture toughness, poor resistance to wear, susceptible to moisture contamination or dehydration during the early stages of the setting reaction. The glass-ionomer cements were first described by Wilson and Kent in 1971 [23], 1972 [24] and at that time, presented a natural extension to the zinc polycarboxylate cements that had become available in the late 1960s. The polycarboxylate cements had evolved from the zinc phosphate cements (prepared by reaction of zinc oxide with phosphoric acid) by the ingenious replacement of the phosphoric acid with poly(acrylic acid). The glass-ionomer cements were immediately seen as a potential replacement for the silicate cements that had been around for some 80 years and which were gradually being ousted by the resin-base composites.

First Generation of Glass-ionomer Cement

Wilson et al made extensive studies on the dental silicate cement and concluded that this cement could not be further improved. They examined cements prepared by mixing dental silicate glass powder with aqueous solutions of various organic acids, including poly(acrylic acid) liquid cement-former. The resultant cement pastes were almost unworkable, set slowly and sluggishly and hydrolytically unstable. Wilson and Kent in 1972 produced a first glass that was high in fluoride (G-200) and that gave usable cement. This cement was originally called as ASPA, an acronym of Alumino-Silicate Polyacrylic Acid. However the first glass ionomer, ASPA I (De trey Division, Dentsply International) set sluggishly, susceptible to moisture while setting and was having very low translucency, resulting in limited use by the clinician.

The solution to the setting problem was discovered by Wilson and Crisp [25], who found that optically active D(+) tartaric acid modified the cement forming reaction, thus improving manipulation, extending working time and sharpening the setting rate. Therefore it is recognized as reaction controlling additive. When added in the liquid in moderate amounts (5%) tartaric acid facilitates the extraction of ions from the glass powder and enables a wider range of glass that can be used for glass ionomers. The introduction of tartaric acid allowed the use of lower fluoride-containing glasses, which are clear or slightly opaque. This refinement of ASPA I was termed as ASPA II and constituted the first practical glass ionomer cement.

The first practical glass ionomer ASPA II used poly(acrylic acid) as a cement-forming liquid. However, solutions of poly(acrylic acid) tend over a period of time to gel when their concentration in water approaches 50% by mass. This is attributed to slow increase in intermolecular bonds. Poly(acrylic acid) chains are flexible and are constantly changing their configurations; when segments of a pair of chains approach each other an intermolecular hydrogen bond can be formed. This is a slow but continuing process. One approach adopted by Wilson and Crisp [26] was to add methyl alcohol to poly(acrylic acid) solution as an agent that inhibits the ordering of structures in solution. Although the gelation of poly(acrylic acid) was prevented, McLean found that the cement stained in the mouth. Crisp and Wilson reasoned that copolymers of acrylic acid would be less regular than the homopolymer of acrylic acid and so less liable to form intermolecular hydrogen bonds. They prepared a copolymer of acrylic acid and itaconic acid, which proved indefinitely stable in a 50% aqueous solution. This copolymer was used in ASPA IV (Table 2.3) [27]. This was the first commercial marketable cement.

Second-generation Glass-ionomer Cement

Water-hardening Glass-ionomer Cement

The conventional glass ionomer is usually supplied as a powder and a polyacid liquid. Unfortunately when the polyacid is present in solution, an increase in either molecular weight or concentration will increase the viscosity of the liquid, making the cement paste progressively more difficult to manipulate. Hence there is a trend using polyacid in solid form for blending with glass ionomer powder. The liquid then for cement formation is either plain water or an aqueous solution of tartaric acid. These cements are called as water mixed or water hardened cements. The main advantages of using this system are the development of low viscosity in the early mixing stages, improved shelf life because there is then no possibility of gelation occurring and improvement in the strength since the molecular weight and polyacid concentration can be increase with this system [22].

Table 2.3. ASPA variants

		Liquid	
ASPA variant	Powder*	Polyacid	Co-monomer
ASPA I	G 200	Acrylic acid Homopolymer, 50% m/m	--------------
ASPA II	G 200	Acrylic acid Homopolymer, 47.5 m/m	Tartaric acid, 50% m/m
ASPA III	G 200	Acrylic acid Homopolymer, 47.5 m/m	Tartaric acid, 4.75% m/m Methanol 5.0 m/m
ASPA IV	G 200	Acrylic acid/itaconic acid copolymer	Tartaric acid, 5.0% m/m

* ASPA Glass G 200: Si 13.3% m/m; Al 13.1% m/m; Ca 17.3% m/m;

	% m/m	atomic fraction
Si	13.3	10.5
Al	13.1	10.8
Ca	17.3	9.6
Na	1.6	1.6
P	2.5	1.8
F	22.7	26.6
O	28.0	39.0

Conventional Glass-ionomer Chemistry

Today conventional glass-ionomer (polyalkenoate) cements are formed by the setting reaction of poly(alkenoic acid)s, i.e. polyelectrolytes, derived from acids such as acrylic acid, methacrylic acid, itaconic acid, maleic acid or 2-butene-1,2,3-tricarboxylic acid (Figure 2.2) with a calcium fluoroaluminosilicate (CaFAlSi) glass powder [28]. Hundreds of glass powder compositions have been studied [27, 29-31]. Even though these powders play a major in establishing the properties of the glass-ionomers, they are given no additional attention in this chapter, since the focus is on polymers. The most useful polyacids, used to date (Figure 2.3) are poly(acrylic acid) (homopolymer of acrylic acid), poly(AA-co-IA) (random copolymer of acrylic acid and itaconic acid) [27] or poly(AA-coMA) (random copolymer of acrylic acid and maleic acid) and to some degree poly(AA-co-MAA) (random copolymer of acrylic acid and methacrylic acid) [32].

There are differences in functionality and acid strength (pK_a) between these polymeric acids. The polymeric acid (polyelectrolyte) in the presence of water attacks the glass powder, releasing calcium and aluminum cations and forming a silica gel area [33]. The poly(alkenoic acid) chains form inter- and intramolecular salt-bridges (Figure 2.4) with the released cations, forming a hard, cross-linked, ceramic-like cement, with some of the molecular structures in the matrix shown in Figure 2.4. This cement undergoes a gradual hardening or setting and maturing process, during which time the ratio of bound to unbound water increases and mechanical properties, such as compressive strength increases gradually with time to a maximum value. The rate of the setting reaction and the final strength of the glass-ionomer cement depend by a number of factors, such as (a) the molecular weight of homopolymer or copolymer, the concentration of water and the powder/liquid ratio [34-36]. As expected the mechanical properties such as toughness, compressive strength, flexural strength and inherent flaw size of the cured compositions increases with the molecular weight of the acidic polymers [35]. (b) the presence or absence of tartaric acid, which shortens the setting time and increases the compressive strength of the cured cement [25,37-39]. (c) the choice of the type of CaFAlSi glass powder (Figure 2.5) and additives [36]. (d) the ratio of the polymeric acid/CaFAlSi glass powder [36].

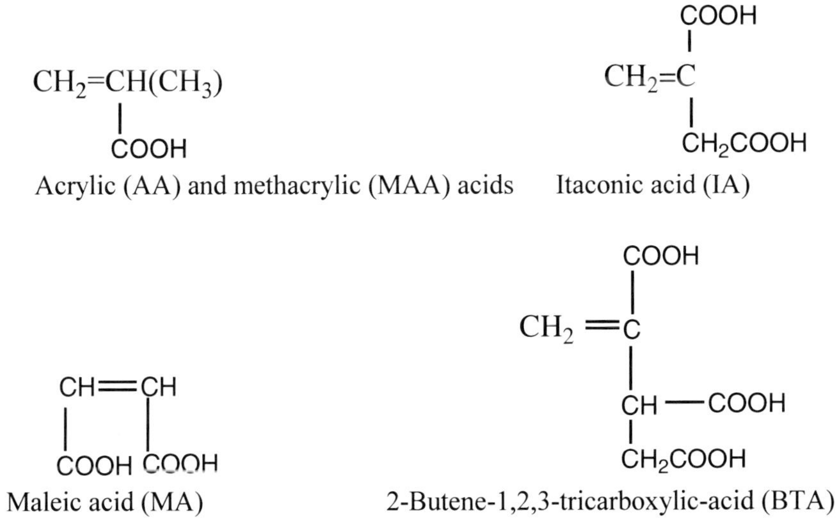

Figure 2.2. Acids studied for preparation of poly(alkenoic acid)s used for producing conventional glass-ionomer cements.

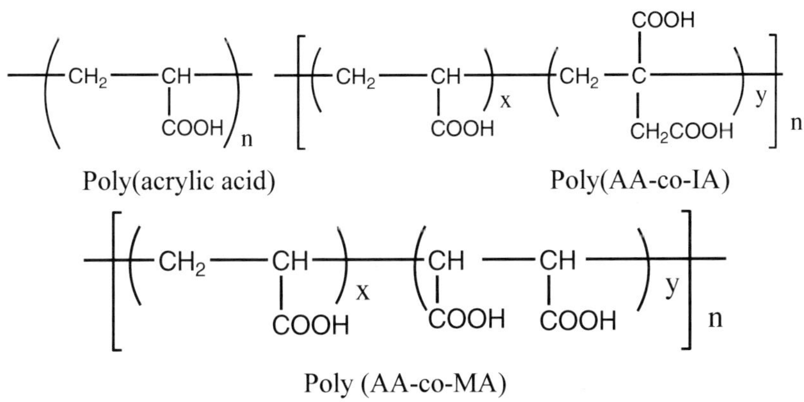

Figure 2.3. Poly(alkenoic acid)s used in glass-ionomer formulations.

The glasses for the glass-ionomer cements contain three main components: silica (SiO_2) and alumina (Al_2O_3) mixed in a flux of calcium fluoride (CaF_2) as shown in Figure 2.5. The composition of the glass is largely restricted to the central region of the phase diagram by the desire to have a translucent glass. The mixture, which also contains sodium and aluminum fluorides and calcium or aluminum phosphates as additional fluxes, is fused at a high temperature and the molten mass is then shock-cooled and finely ground to a powder before use. The particle size of the powder is dependent upon its intended application. For filling materials the maximum particle size is 50 μm, while for the luting and lining materials it is reduced to less than 20 μm.

The rate of release of ions from the glass, which is an important factor in determining the setting characteristics, the solubility and the release of fluoride, is a function of the type of glass employed. The glass also plays a major role in the aesthetics of the restoration, as this is dependent on both the refractive index of the glass and the presence of pigments within it [4].

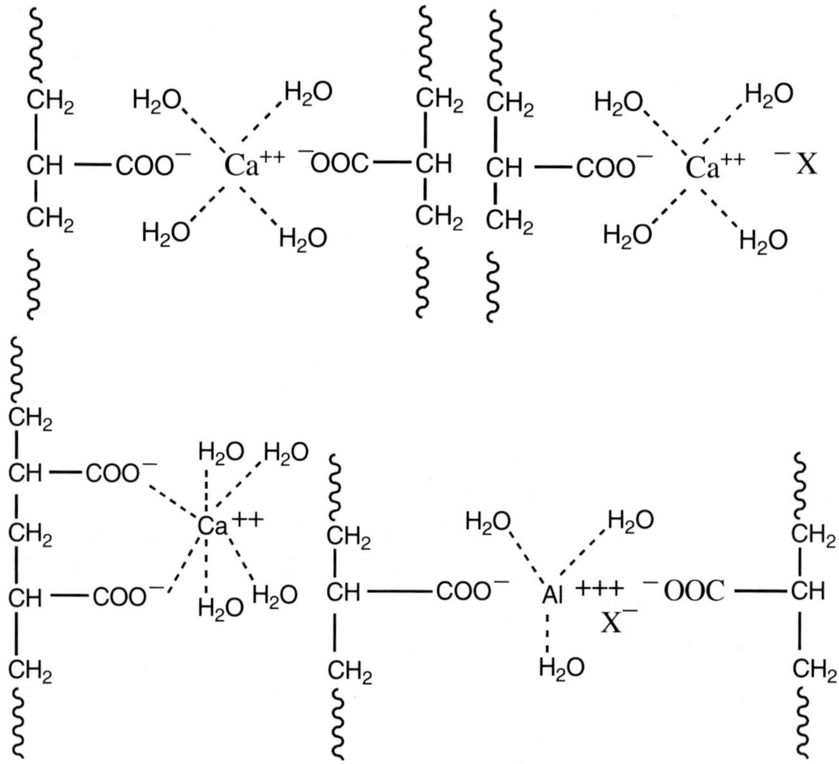

Figure 2.4. Possible inter- and intramolecular salt bridges between the poly(alkenoic acid) and the released cationsCa^{2+} or Al^{3+}, where X represents OH$^-$ or F$^-$ anions.

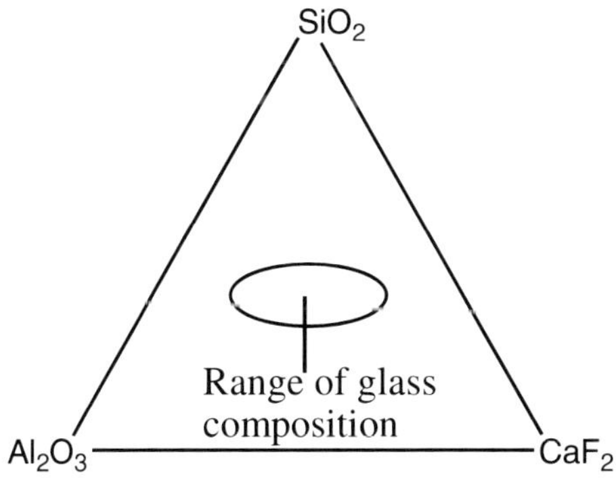

Figure 2.5. Composition of glass used in glass-ionomer cements.

2.4.3. Reinforced Glass-ionomer Cements

The conventional glass ionomer cement has been used successfully for the esthetic filling of cavities subjected to low stresses, for example, the restorationof class V erosion lesions, class III restorations and for the filling or sealing of pit and fissures.However the low tensile strength of existing formulations (7-14 MPa) makes the cement unsuitable for use in high stress sites, such as class IIrestorations, particularly where there is lack of support from the cavity wall. The cement must be improved in strength if it is to find a wider range of publications [22].They did so by

It was Wilson and Prosser who first reported attempts to improve the strength of glass-ionomers by reinforcement [40]. They did so by the incorporation of metal fibers and flakes into the setting cement, an approach that was successful in improving the flexural strength. However, there were problems in that these cements showed a correspondingly poor wear resistance and a greater tendency to fracture. Since this early work, two approaches have been employed to reinforce these cements: (a) the incorporation of powdered metal, such as silver alloy [41] from conventional amalgam alloy and (b) the fusing of the metal typically silver with a reactive glass powder to make a sintered ceramic-metal powder known as a *cermet* and using this powder to form cements by reaction with a polyacid [42].Cermets for glass-ionomers have also been made from gold [43] but this form has not been manufactured commercially. Clinically, metal containing glass-ionomers and cermet have been used for a variety of purposes. In addition to core built-up prior to placement of crowns they have been used for Class I and Class II restorations in primary teeth. A number of studies have confirmed their effectiveness in these applications and their cariostatic properties in clinical use [44,45].

Materials other than metal or cermet powders have been used in attempts to reinforce glass-ionomers. Prosser at al. [36] for example employed metal fibers. Unfortunately these cements were more prone to wear than the unfilled cement, hence this approach was abandoned. Others investigated the use of both carbon and alumino-silicate fibers to reinforce glass-ionomers, as a possible route to the development of glass-ionomer cements for use in orthopaedic surgery. This led to increased Young's modulus and increased flexural strength, but unfortunately these rein forced cements proved difficult to mix [46]. Finally Nicholson et al. studied the inclusion of finely divided hydroxyapatite into glass ionomers. The effects of this inclusion were found to vary with the glass used. [47].

2.4.4. Resin-modified Glass-ionomer Cements

Resin-modified glass-ionomer cements are hybrid cements which cure or harden by two mechanisms, i.e, partly via an acid-base reaction and partly via a free-radical photopolymerization. The material is presented either as a powder-liquid system or in capsule form. In the first case the powder consists of a radiopaque fluoro-alumino-silicate glass and a photoactive liquid kept in the dark bottle to protect it from ambient light. The liquid composition varies from product to product, but in general it is an aqueous solution of hydrophilic monomers, such as 2-hydroxyethyl methacrylate (HEMA) or Bis-GMA which copolymerize with the methacrylate functionalized polyacid to give a highly cross-linked organic matrix [48-50].

The acid-base reaction is essentially the same as for the glass-ionomer cements and is initiated when the powder and the liquid are mixed. The material differs from other glass-ionomer cements in that this reaction is much slower, giving a considerably longer working time. The rapid set is provided by the light curing of HEMA or Bis-GMA and additional crosslinking through the reaction of HEMA or Bis-GMA with the pendant methacrylate groups of polyacid.

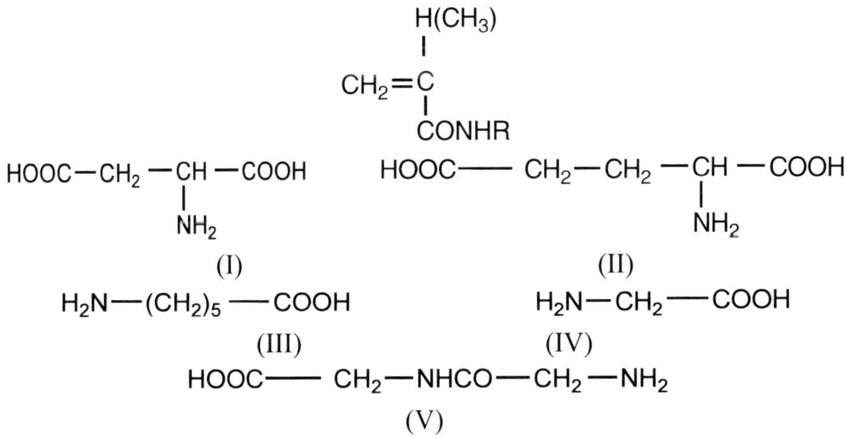

Figure 2.6. N-acryloyl and N-methacryloyl substituted amino acid monomers RNH- comes from aspartic acid (I), glutamic acid (II), 6-aminocaproic acid (III), glycine (IV) or glycylglycine (V) etc.

2.4.5. New Conventional Glass-ionomers

One of the problems with chemically cured poly(acrylic acid) or acrylic acid copolymers with itaconic acid or maleic acid (Fig.2.3) lies in the direct of very close attachment of the carboxylic groups to the polymeric backbone, resulting in a very rigid matrix. Wilson et al. suggest that not all the carboxyl groups of poly(acrylic acid) are converted to carboxylate groups during the course of the reaction. Their studies have shown that very few inter- or intramolecular Al^{3+} tricarboxylate (Figure 2.6) complexes (salt bridges) are formed, which is understandable in view of steric requirements [28]. About the mid 90s, a new family of polyacids (polyelectrolytes) with carboxylic groups tethered various distances from the polymer backbone, via flexible side chains attached randomly along the polymer backbone, was studied [51]. The monomers used to modify the acrylic or methacrylic acid are shown in Figure 2.6.

The removal of reactive functionalities from direct attachment polymer backbones via the use of various spacer groups, allows greater access for reaction, especially on a rigid polymer backbone. The spacer moiety or tethering unit serves to dissociate steric hindrance of the polymer main chain from the assembly, while not affecting the reactivity of the spacer linked functionality. The functionality, in this case a –COOH group, has more freedom to undergo reaction. The spacer linked functionality has much greater degree of freedom from constraint by the polymer backbone since the rigid polymer chain cannot bent or flex sufficiently to make most of the –COOH groups available for reaction. At the same time, however, the length and type of spacer group can be used to influence changes in hydrophilicity, conformation in solution, viscosity and solubility of the polymers. It is also expected that –COOH groups tethered to the polymer backbone, with various lengths of spacers moieties, will have much greater degrees of freedom to react with Ca^{2+} and Al^{3+} ions liberated from the reactive glass, resulting in enhanced filler-polymer interaction, more complete salt-bridge formation between three $-COO^-$ anion residues and one Al^{3+} cation and enhanced homogeneity in the matrix [28].The spacer moiety or tethering unit serves to dissociate steric hindrance of the polymer main chain from the assembly, while not affecting the reactivity of the spacer linked functionality [52-54]. Thus tethering amino acids to the polymer backbone provides more freedom and less steric hindrance, availability of different types of carboxylic acid residues and different pH values, promoting more salt-bridge formation [55].This approach was found to improve mechanical properties of the formulated glass-ionomers [56].

Polyelectrolytes Containing Amide Groups

The amido-acid monomers prepared for tethering different types of acid groups,various distance of the polymer backbone of acrylic acid (AA) or methacrylic acid (MA) and itaconic acid (IA) copolymers are shown in Figure 2.6. The use of amido-acid monomers in the production of new polyelectrolytes for glass-ionomer formulation showed that the reaction product of glutamic acid with methacryloyl chloride known as MGA is the best to use, since reaction of glutamic acid with methacryloyl chloride gives good yields of crystalline MGA [28].

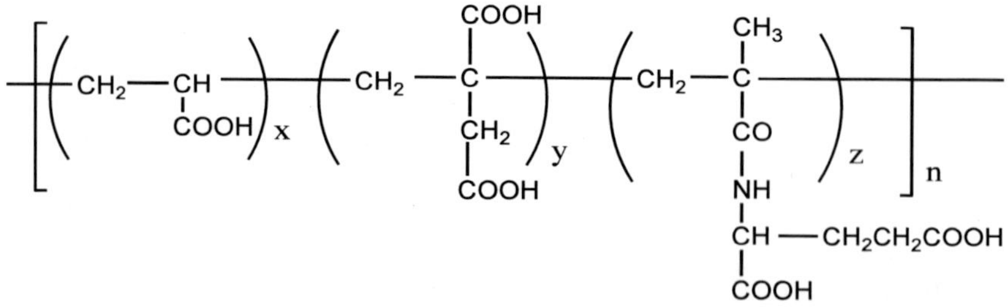

Figure 2.7. Copolymer of AA, IA and MGA.

AA, IA and MGA were copolymerized in water with free radicals initiators to produce copolymers $AA_xIA_yMGA_z$ having the structure shown in Figure 2.7. Copolymers having x/y/z ratios of 7/3/3 and 8/1/1 showed improved properties.

Polyelectrolytes Containing N-Vinylpyrrolidone

Poly (acrylic acid) first used to formulate glass-ionomers, was found to be unstable in aqueous solutions at elevated molecular weights, that is the solution forms a gel. Thus, itaconic acid or maleic acid was incorporated into the polymer backbone to provide disorder enabling formulators to have stabile aqueous solutions of the copolymers with ca. 50% solids. It was theorized that a fair mumber of the AA,IA OR MA, residues could be replaced in the copolymer backbone by NVP, maintaining water solubility for the copolymer and providing a new path to explore for generating improved performance glass ionomers [57-59]. NVP is readily polymerized with free radical initiators giving a non-ionogenic, water soluble, non toxic polymer.

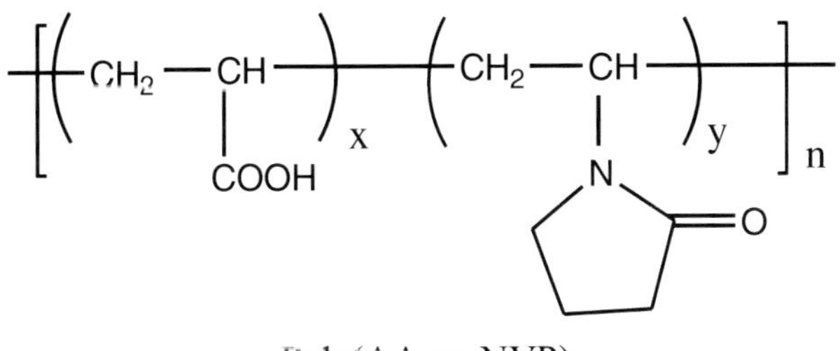

Poly(AA-co-NVP)

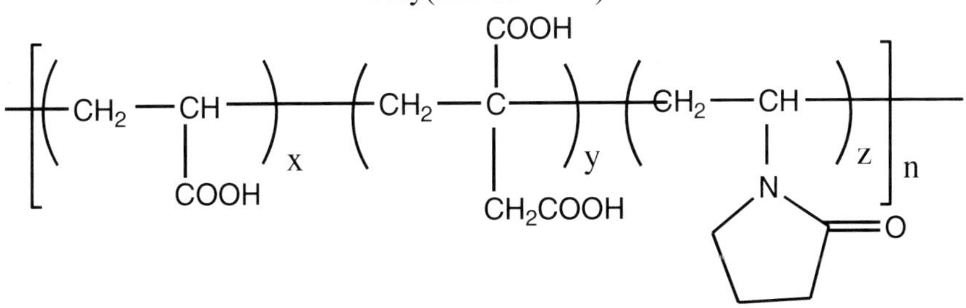

Poly(AA-co-IA-co-NVP)

Figure 2.8. Random copolymers Poly(AA-co-NVP) and Poly(AA-co-IA-co-NVP).

Even though the NPV polymer is easily soluble in water, studies have shown that water is not a thermodynamically good solvent for the homopolymer [60]. The solubility is probably due to some degree of compensation between the strong hydrogen bonding capability, that is hydrogen bonding between the cyclic amide group and water and hydrophobic interactions that exist between water and the NVP polymer backbone and cyclic methylene groups. It is plausiblethat the strong hydrogen bonding can lead to polymer swelling that is expansion of the polymeric coils, while the hydrophobic interactions could bring about compression of the coils. Whatever that case, the NVP homopolymer is known to strongly absorb water [60], with the absorption center being the amide group. In contrast to water soluble poly(acrylic acid) or poly(methacrylic acid), NVP homopolymer does not precipitate from aqueous solution without salts, even after heating to 100°C. The latter suggests the hydrophilic interactions, which would promote aggregation, do not over compensate for the strong hydrophilic nature of the NVP polymer, which result from strong hydrogen bonding. These properties make NVP a good candidate to try and exploit in the development of polyelectrolytes for application in glass-ionomer formulation [28].

A poly(AA-co-NVP) (Figure 2.8) was evaluated in glass-ionomer formulation. Aqueous solution (50% solids) of copolymer which contained 75% AA was blended with a glass powder used in a commercial glass-ionomer (Fuji II). Mixing of the glass powder with a 50% aqueous solution of copolymer poly(AA-co-NVP) at the same powder/liquid ratio (2.7/1) recommended for the commercial glass-ionomer Fuji II, placing the mixture in suitable mold, curing, conditioning and testing produced a glass-ionomer with higher compression strength, flexure strength and diametral tensile strength than commercial glass-ionomer used as control. These preliminary results from evaluating the poly(AA-co-NVP) gave support to the concept that there might be an opportunity to use NVP to develop new water soluble copolymers for improved performance glass-ionomers [61].

Also to shed further light on the possible use of NVP, a random copolymer poly(AA-co-IA-co-NVP) was prepared (Figure 2.8) with 7/3/1 ratio of monomer units respectively.

The experimental glass-ionomer based on poly(AA-co-IA-co-NVP) random copolymer showed improved physical and mechanical properties compared with the commercial glass-ionomer Fuji II which is based on poly(AA-co-IA) random copolymer.

In the efford to determine what the x,y,z ratio should be for poly(AA-co-IA-co-NVP) (Fig.2.8) and what the copolymer molecular weight should be to obtain the optimum properties sixteen copolymers were prepared having different AA/IA/NVP monomer ratios and different molecular weights [62]. Flexural strength (FS) was selected as the primary mechanical property to try to optimize, since FS is one of the properties needing significant improvement. Prosser et al. [36] suggested that the most appropriate measure of the strength of glass-ionomer cements was FS, since a material could fail by separation of the planes of atoms, (i.e. tensile failure) or by slipping of the planes of atoms (i.e. shear failure). The FS test is a collective measurement of three types of stresses, simultaneously, i.e. tensile at one surface of the specimen beam compression at the other surface and shear in the direction which is parallel to the load stress. [36]. The measurement of FS for sixteen copolymers showed that the molar ratio of 7/1/3 (AA/IA/NVP) was near optimum for the copolymer to have the highest FS value [59].

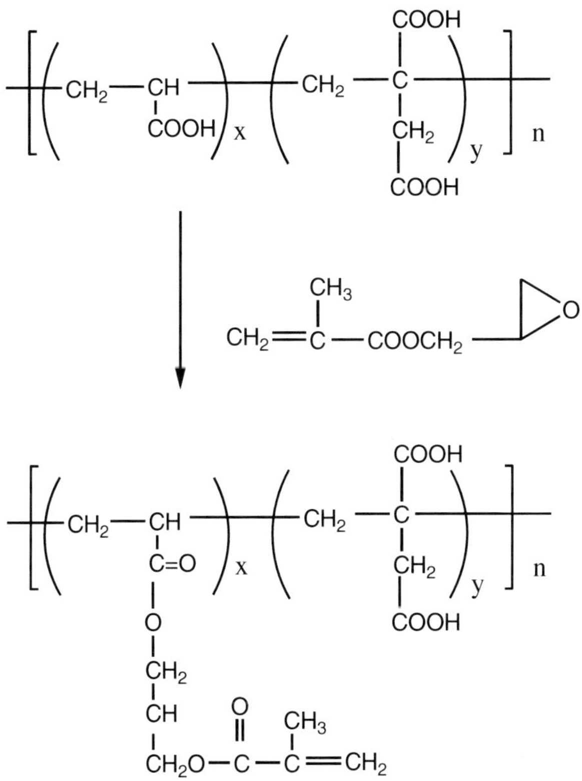

Figure 2.9. Reaction of poly(AA-co-IA) with glycidyl methacrylate for producing a light cured glass-ionomer.

2.4.6. New Visible Light-cured Glass-ionomers

Visible light-cured glass-ionomers (VLC) were originally developed as hybrids of self curing (classical) glass-ionomers and resin composites [48]. To achieve a stable solution of the aqueous and organic components, the water soluble 2-hydroxyethyl methacrylate (HEMA) was used. HEMA acts both as a co-solvent and a free radical light-cured monomer. Very soon, after the latter initial discovery, alternative monomers and concepts were used to make cements of this type. The concepts included the use of copolymers in which polymerizable side chains were attached to the main polymer backbone via reactions of a significant number of the pendant carboxylic groups of the backbone with vinyl monomers such as glycidyl methacrylate [63] (Figure 2.9] or 2-isocyanatoethyl methacrylate (IEM) [64,65] as shown in Figure 2.10.

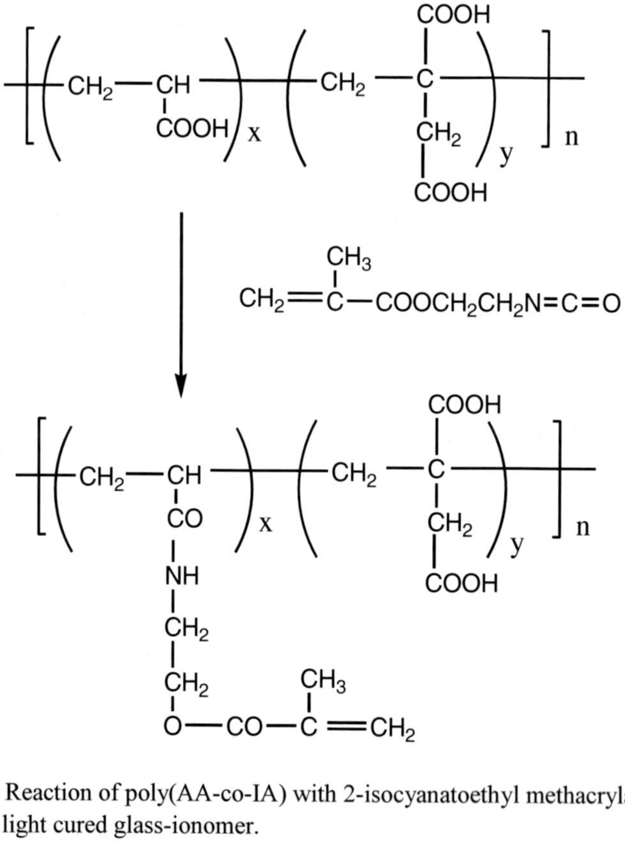

Figure 2.10. Reaction of poly(AA-co-IA) with 2-isocyanatoethyl methacrylate for producing a light cured glass-ionomer.

Current light cured glass-ionomers consist of a complex mixture of components. These are (i) poly(acrylic acid) or a modified poly(acrylic acid) (ii) a photocurable monomer such as hydroxyethyl methacrylate (HEMA) or a photocurable side chaingrafted on to the poly(acrylic acid) (iii) an ion-leachable glass and (iv) water. Consequently they set by a number of competing reactions to give complex structures.

The initial setting reaction is the photochemical polymerization. Depending on the precise details of the formulation, this process is either a copolymerization of the HEMA with the polymer side chain or homopolymerization of the functional groups in the side chains. Subsequently, the acid-base reactions typical of glass-ionomers take place. This process is designed to be slower than in conventional glass-ionomers; it is also probably impeded by the development of photopolymrized network. These reactions may be assumed to be as follows [66,67].

1. Decomposition of the glass under the influence of the polyacid, leading to release of Ca^{2+} ions and Al^{3+} species, these latter probably being in the form of complex oxy-anions containing several aluminium atoms.
2. Rapid reaction of the Ca^{2+} ions with the polyacid chains, followed by slower reaction of Al^{3+} species gradually released from the anionic complex.
3. Gradual hydration of the silicate fragments released in step 1 to yield a matrix of increased strength and greater resistance to desiccation

LITERATURE

[1] Combe, E.C.; Burke, F.J.T; Douglas, W.H. *Dental Biomaterials.* Boston: Kluwer Academic Publishers; 1999.

[2] Craig, R.G. Restorative Dental Materials. 10th ed. St Louis, Missouri: Mosby-Year book, Inc. 1997.

[3] http://www.doctorspiller.com/denture_relines.htm

[4] Van Noort, R. *Introduction to Dental Materials.* 2nd ed. Edinburgh: Mosby, 2002.

[5] Kasuga, Y.; Akiba, N.; Minakuchi, S.; Uchida, T.; Matsushita,N.; Hishimoto, M.; and Hayakawa, I. Development of Soft Denture Lining

Material Containing Fluorinated Monomers. *J Jpn Prosthodont Soc* 52 : 183-188, 2008

[6] Braden, M.; Clarke, R.L.; Nicholson, J.; Parker, S. *Polymeric Dental Materials.* Berlin Heidelberg: Springer-Verlag 1997.

[7] Van Handel, AB. (1974). *US Patent* 3785 054

[8] May, P.; Guerra, LR (1981). *US Patent* 4251 215.

[9] Braden, M. (1970). Tissue Conditioners: II. Rheologic Properties. *J Dent Res* 49, 496-501.

[10] Braden, M. (1971). The rheology of dental tissue conditioners. *Rheol Acta* 10, 86-90.

[11] Braden, M.; Causton, BE (1971). Tissue Conditioners: III. Water Immersion Characteristics. *J Dent Res* 50, 1544-47.

[12] Jones, DW.; Sutow, EJ.; Hall, GG.; Tobin, WM.; Graham, BS. (1988). Dental soft polymers: plasticizer composite and leachability *Dent Mater* 4, 1-7

[13] Graham, BS.; Jones, DW.; Sutow, EJ (1989). Clinical implications of resilient denture lining material research. Part I: Flexibility and elasticity. *J Prosthet Dent* 1989;62:421-8.

[14] Herman F. Mark, Norbert Bikales, Charles G. Overberger, Georg Menges. (1986). Encyclopedia of Polymer Science and Engineering, Volume 4, *Composities, Fabrication to Die Design,* 2nd Edition.Wiley. NJ. p. 704.

[15] Braden, M. (1988). Some aspects on the chemistry and physics of dental resins. *Advances in Dental Research.* 2 (1), 93-97.

[16] http://en.wikipedia.org/wiki/Dental_cement

[17] Wilson, A.D. (1982). The nature of the zinc polycarboxlyate cement matrix, *J Biomed Mater Res,* 16, 549-557.

[18] Nicholson, J.W.; Brookman, P.J.; Lacy, O,M.; Sayers, G.S.; Wilson, A.D.(1988). A study of the nature and formation of zinc polyacrylate cement using Fourier transform infrared spectroscopy. *J Biomed Mater Res,* 22, 623-31.

[19] Nicholson, J.W. The Chemistry of Medical and Dental Materials. (2002). *RSC Materials Monographs, series editor Connor,* J.A. Cambridge, UK.

[20] Nicholson, J.W.; Hawkins, Wasson, E.A. (1993). A study of the structure of zinc polycarboxylate dental cements. *J Mater Sci Mater Med* 4, 32-35.

[21] Nicholson, J.W.; Wilson, A.D. (2000). The effect of storage in aqueous solutions on glass-ionomer and zinc polycarboxylate dental cements. *J Mater Sci Mater Med,* 11, 357-360

[22] Nagaraja Upadhya, P.; Kishore, G. (2005). Glass Ionomer Cement-The Different Generations. Trends Biomater. *Artif. Organs,* 18 (2), 158-165.

[23] Wilson, A.D.; Kent, B.E. (1971) The glass-ionomer cement, a new translucent dental filling material. *J Appl Chem Biotechnol,* 21, 313-318.

[24] Wilson, A.D.; Kent, B.E. (1972). A new translucent cement for dentistry. The glass-ionomer cement. *Br Dent J,* 132-135.

[25] Crisp, S.; Wilson, A. D. (1976). "Reactions in Glass-Ionomer Cements. V. Effect of Incorporating Tartaric Acid in the Cement Liquid,"]. *Dent. Res.* 55, 1023-1031.

[26] Crisp, S.; Wilson, A. D. (1974) Reactions in glass ionomer cements: III. The precipitation reaction.]. *Dent. Res.* 53,1420-1424.

[27] Crisp, S.; Ferner, A.J.; Lewis, B.G.; Wilson, A.D. (1975). Properties of improved glass-ionomer cement formulations. *Journal of Dentistry* 3, 125-130.

[28] Culbertson, B.M. (2001). Glass-ionomer dental restoratives. *Prog. Polym. Sci.* 26, 577-604.

[29] McLean, Wilson, A.D. (1977). The Clinical Development of the Glass Ionomer Cements. 1. Formulations and Properties, *Aust Dent J,* 22, 31-36.

[30] Kent, B.E.; Lewis, B.G.; Wilson, A.D. (1979). Glass Ionomer Cement Formulations: I. The Preparation of Novel Fluoroaluminosilicate Glasses High in Fluorine. *J Dent Res,* 58, 1607-1619

[31] Crisp, S.; Kent, B.E.; Lewis, B.G.; Ferner, A.J.; Wilson, A.D.(1980). Glass-ionomer Cement Formulations. II. *The Synthesis of Novel Polycarboxylic J Dent Res,* 59, 1055-1063

[32] Schmidt, W.; Purmann, R.; Jochum, P.; Gasser, O.(1981). *Eur Patent Appl* 24,056.

[33] Wasson, E.A.; Nicholson, J.W. (1990). A study of the relationship between setting chemistry and properties of modified glass poly(alkenoate) cements. *Br Polym J* 23:179 183.

[34] Crisp, S.; Lewis, B.G.; Wilson, A.D. (1977). Characterization of Glass-ionomer Cements.3. Effect of Polyacid Concentration on the Physical Properties, *J Dent* 5:51-56, 1977.

[35] Wilson, A.D.; Crisp, S.; Abel, G. (1977). Characterization of Glass-ionomer Cements. 4. Effect of Molecular Weight on Physical Properties, *Journal of Dentistry,* 5(2): 117–120.

[36] Prosser, H.J.; Powis, D.R.; Wilson, A.D. (1986). Glass-ionomer cements of improved flexural strength. *J Dent Res* 65:146-148.

[37] Prosser, H.J.; Jerome, S.M.; Wilson, A.D. (1982). The Effect of Additives on the Setting Properties of a Glass-Ionomer Cement *J Dent Res* 61, 1195-1198.

[38] Prosser, H.J.; Richards, C.P.; Wilson, A.D. (1982). The Role of Tartaric Acid in Glass-Ionomer Cements,*J Biomed Mater Res*, 16, 431-445.

[39] Cook, W.D. (1983). Dental polyelectrolyte cements III. Effect of additives on their rheology. *Biomaterials,* 4, 85-88

[40] Wilson, A.D.; Prosser, H.J.; (1984) A survey of inorganic and polyelectrolyte cements. *British Dental Journal,* 157, 279-282.

[41] Simmons, J.J. (1983). The miracle mixture: glass-ionomer and alloy powder. *Texas Dental Journal* 100, 6-12.

[42] McLean, J.W. Gasser, O. (1985). Glass cermet cements. Quintessence International 16, 333-343.

[43] McLean, J.W. (1990). Cermet cements *Journal of the American Dental Association,* 120, 43-47.

[44] Hickel, R.; Voss, A.; (1990). Clinical evaluation of glass-ionomer cement and amalgam restorations in primary molars. *Journal of Dentistry for Children,* 57, 184-188.

[45] Hung, T.W.; Richardson A.S. (1990). Evaluation of glass-ionomer silver cermet restorations in primary molars: one year results. *Journal of the Canadian Dental Association,* 56 239-240.

[46] Oldfield, C.W.B.; Ellis, B.; (1991). Fibrous reinforcement of glass-ionomer cements. *Clinical Materials,* 7, 313-323.

[47] Nicholson, J.W.; Hawkins, S.; Smith, J.E. (1993). The incorporation of hydroxyapatite into glass polyalkenoate ("glass-ionomer" cements: a preliminary study. *J Mater Sci., Mater in Medicine* 4, 418-421.

[48] Antonucci JM, McKinney JE, Stansbury JW (1988). Resin modified glass-ionomer dental cements field of the invention. US Patent Application 7,160,856. Springfield, VA: *National Technical Information Service.*

[49] Mitra SB (1989). Photocurable ionomer cement systems. *European Patent Application* No. 88312127.9, publication No. 0323120.

[50] Smith, D.C. (1990). Composition and characteristics of glass ionomer cements. *J Am Dent Assoc,* 120:20-2.

[51] Kao, E.C.; Culbertson, B.M.; Xie, D. (1996). Preparation of glass-ionomer cement using N-acryloyl-substituted amino acid monomers: evaluation of physical properties. *Dent Mater* 12, 44-51.

[52] Finklemen, H.; Ringsdorf, H.; Wendorff, J.H. Model considerations and examples of enantiotropic liquid crystalline polymers. *Makromol Chem,* 1978; 179, 273.

[53] Barbucci, R.; Casolaro, M.; Magnani, A. (1989). Vinyl polymers containing amido and carboxylic groups as side substituents II. Thermodynamic and FT-IR spectroscopic studies for the protonation of poly(N-acryloyl-glycine) and poly(N-acryloyl-6-caproic acid). *Die Makromolekulare Chemie*, 190, 2627-2638.

[54] Barbucci, R.; Casolaro, M.; Magnani, A. Roncalini, C. (1991). Different protonation behavior of two poly(methacrylic acid) derivatives containing N-acylglycine and N-acyl-β-alanine residues: thermodynamic and FT-IR studies *Macromolecules,* 24, 1249-52.

[55] Ouyang, Z.; Sneckenberger, S.K.; Kao, E.C.; Culbertson, B.M.; Jagodzinski, P.W. (1991). New Method for Monitoring the Reaction of Glass-Ionomer Cements: A Spectroscopic Study of the Effects of Polyacid Structure on the Decomposition of Calcium Aluminosilicate Glasses. *Appl Spectrosc,* 53, 297-301.

[56] Culbertson, B.M.; Xie, D.; Thakur, A. (1999). New matrix resins for glass polyalkenates or glass-ionomers with pendant amino acid residues, *J. M. S., Pure Appl. Chem.,* 1999; A36(5-6): 681-696. *J Macromol Sci., Pure Appl Chem,* A36, 681-96.

[57] Xie, D.; Culbertson, B.M.; Wang, G. (1998). Microhardness of *N*-vinylpyrrolidone modified glass-ionomers cements. *J Macromol Sci, Pure Appl Chem,* A35, 547-61.

[58] Xie, D.; Culbertson, B.M.; Johnston, W.M. (1998). Improved Flexural Strength of N-vinylpyrrolidone Modified Acrylic Acid Copolymers for Glassionomers, *J Macromol Sci, Pure Appl Chem,* A35, 1615-29.

[59] Xie, D.; Culbertson, B.M.; Johnston, W.M. (1998). Formulations of light-curable glass-ionomer cements containing N-vinylpyrolidone. J Macromol Sci, *Pure Appl Chem,* A35, 1631-50.

[60] Levy, G.B.; Frank, H.P.(1955). Determination of molecular weight of polyvinylpyrrolidone. II. *J Polym Sci* 17, 247-254.

[61] Xie, D.; Culbertson, B.M. (1996). Water soluble N-vinylpyrrolidone copolymers for improved glass-ionomer systems. *J Dent Res* 75, 298-343.

[62] Culbertson, B.M.; Xie, D.; Thakur, A. (1998). Amino acid functionalized ionomeric materials in biomedical applications. *Macromol Symp,* 131,11-18.
[63] Engelbrecht, J. (1989) Polymerizable cement mixtures. *US Patent* 4,872,935.
[64] Mitra, S.B.; Mitra S. (1992) Universal water-based medical and dental cement. *US Patent* 5,154,762.
[65] Mitra, S.B.(1992). Photocurable ionomer cement systems. *US Patent* 5,130,347.
[66] Nicholson, J.W.; Anstice H.M. (1994). The development of modified glass-ionomer cements for dentistry. *Trends Polym Sci,* 2, 272-8.
[67] Anstice H.M.; Nicholson, J.W. (1992). Studies on the structure of light cured glass ionomer cement. *J Mater Sci Mater Med*, 3, 447–451.

Chapter 3

POLYMERIC DENTAL RESTORATIVE MATERIALS

3.1. POLYMERIC COMPOSITES

Dental amalgam has traditionally been employed as material for tooth cavity filling for about 200 years and is still in many ways a suitable restorative material. Its advantages are strength, relatively easy clinical handling and low cost. Disadvantages are lack of adhesive properties to tooth substance and its non-aesthetic character. Dental amalgam is an alloy of mercury (50%), silver (30%), tin, copper and zinc. It is made by dissolving the solid metals in the liquid mercury. However the use of this material is controversial because of esthetic problems, eventual toxicity, environmental pollution by mercury etc [1]. Dental polymer composites were introduced commercially for restoring the anterior teeth in the mid-1960s and their introduction was one of the most significant contributions to dentistry in the last century. Since their commercial introduction their characteristics such as the physical properties, manipulative qualities, durability and wear resistance have improved remarkably. As a result they are widely used instead of amalgam. Composites make up for the weak points of amalgam, such as toxicity from mercury content, corrosion and low adhesive property. In addition composites have a better aesthetic property than amalgam. The scope of their applications has expanded continuously from small anterior restorations to large posterior restorations and even fixed partial dentures [2, 3].

Physical-chemical requirements for dental monomers

- High rate of photopolymerization and cross-linking properties
- Low volume shrinkage or expansion during polymerization
- Optimal mechanical properties and wear resistance
- T_g above 60°C and low water-uptake of the formed polymer
- Excellent resistance to oral conditions
- High light and coloration stability of the formed polymer
- Storage stability in the presence of dental fillers and additives
- Low oral toxicity, no mutagenic or carcinogenic effect

Figure 3.1. Basic requirements for monomers used in dental composites.

3.1.1. Composition of Dental Polymer Composites

A composite as the name implies is a mixture of two or more components, in which the individual components retain their physical identity. More importantly a composite material is a multiphase material that exhibits properties of the constituent phases in such a way as to produce a material with a better combination of properties than could be realized by any of the component phases. The dental polymer composites have three major components:

- An organic polymer matrix
- An inorganic filler
- A coupling agent

3.1.1.1. Polymeric Matrix-initiators

At present the polymer matrix of dental composites are mainly based on a mixture of dimethacrylates and have to fulfill a number of basic requirements with regard to the reactivity, stability or toxicity of the monomers used and the properties (strength, stiffness, stability) of the formed polymer network (Figure 3.1).

In currently used dental composites the polymer matrix is based on the following dimethacrylates, 2,2-bis[4-2-hydroxy-3-(methacryloxy)propyl] phenyl]propane (Bis-GMA), ethoxylated Bis-GMA (Bis-EMA), 1,6-bis-[2-methacryloyloxyethoxycarbonylamino]-2,4,4-trimethylhexane (UDMA), decanediol dimethacrylate (D_3MA) or triethyleneglycol dimethacrylate (TEGDMA), are used (Figure 3.2) [2, 4-7].

All these monomers have a double bond in common, which is opened up to allow the monomer to bond to a neighboring monomer. This process of preparing polymers from monomers is called addition polymerization. The process of addition polymerization involves three stages, initiation, propagation and termination. The initiation involves first the formation of free radicals usually by decomposition of peroxide. The peroxide commonly used in dental materials is benzoyl peroxide (BPO). Under appropriate conditions a molecule of BPO can yield two free radicals (Figure 3.3):

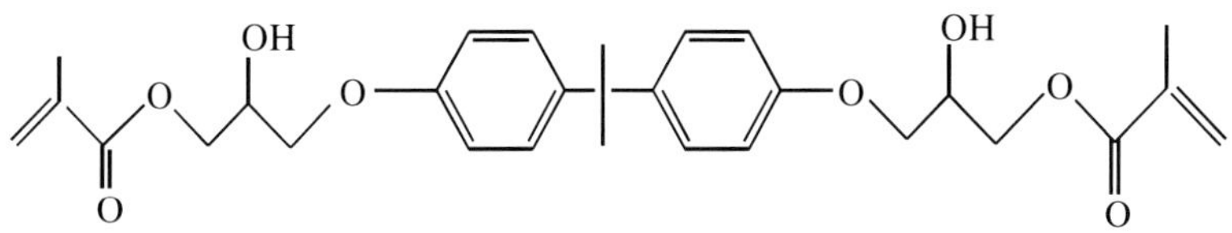

Bis-GMA

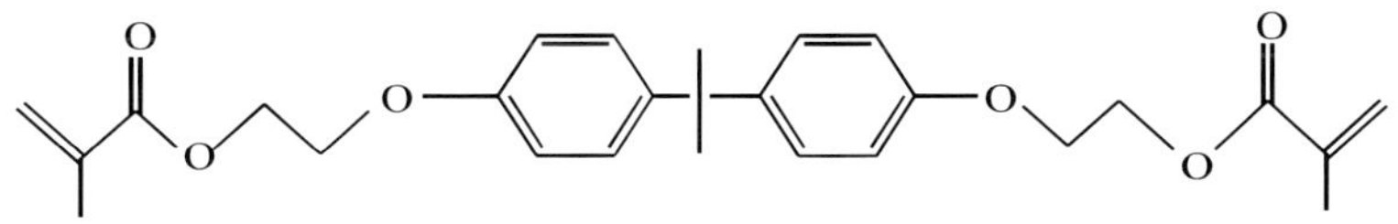

Bis-EMA

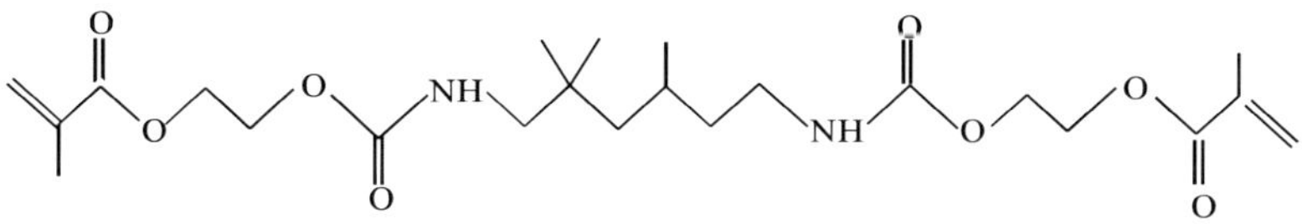

UDMA

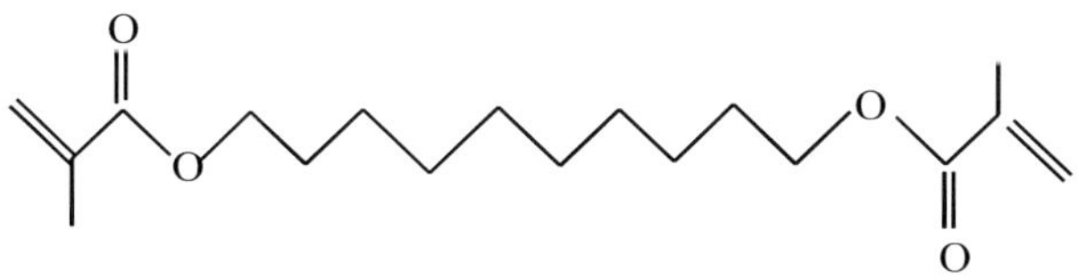

D_3MA

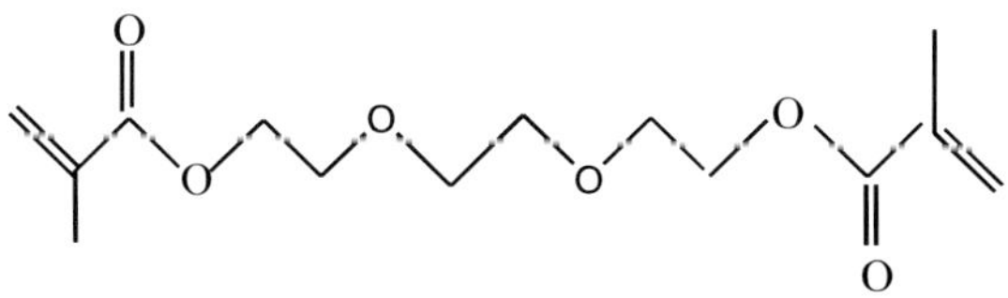

TEGDMA

Figure 3.2. Structure of dimethacrylates frequently used in dental polymer composites.

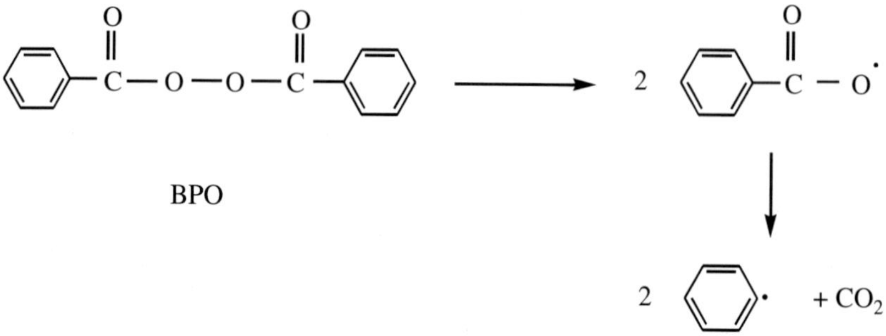

Figure 3.3. Mechanism of thermal decomposition of benzoyl peroxide (BPO).

The decomposition of the peroxide is achieved by the heat, by the use of chemical compounds or the light. When the peroxide heated above 65°C it decomposes as shown above. The peroxide can also be activated when brought into contact with a tertiary amine such as N,N-dimethyl-p-toluidine (DMT), 4-(*N,N*-dimethylamino)phenethyl alchohol (DMPOH), 4-(*N,N*-dimethylamino)phenylacetic acid (DMAPAA) and ethyl 4-(dimethylamino)benzoate (EDMAB) (Figure 3.4) [8-11].

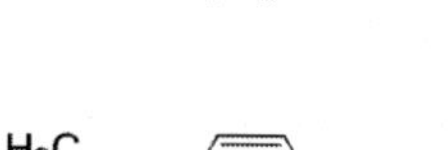

DMT

N,N-dimethyl-p-toluidine

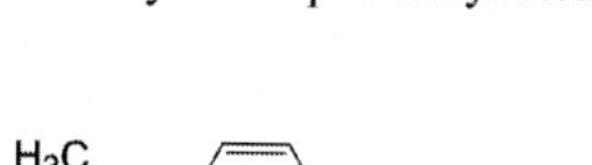

DMPOH

4-N,N-dimethylaminophenethyl alchohol

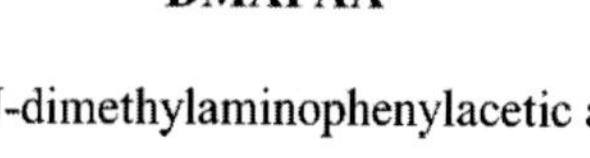

DMAPAA

4-N,N-dimethylaminophenylacetic acid

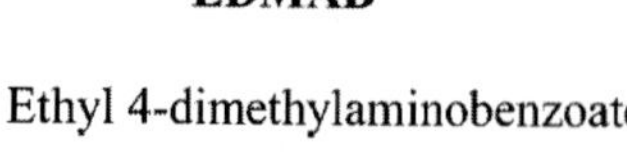

EDMAB

Ethyl 4-dimethylaminobenzoate

Figure 3.4. Chemical structure of the para-substituted derivatives of dimethylaniline, used as co-initiators with benzoyl peroxide.

In our lab the free radical homopolymerization of Bis-GMA, UDMA and TEGDMA by a BPO/amine redox couple were studied by differential scanning calorimetry (DSC) [8]. As amine para-substituted N, N-dimethyl aniline derivatives DMT, DMPOH, DMAPAA and EDMAB were used. Amines with electron –donating para-substituents such as $–CH_3$, $-CH_2CH_2OH$, or $–CH_2COOH$ was found to be efficient co-initiators for polymerization at 37°C. On the contrary the amine with the electron-withdrawing para-substituent $COOCH_2CH_3$ could not initiate polymerization at 37°C, but only at higher temperatures. The kinetic parameters of polymerization are strongly affected also by the chemical structure of the monomer. UDMA showed the highest value for the maximum polymerization rate followed by Bis-GMA and TEGDMA. TEGDMA showed the highest degree of final conversion (ca 70%) followed by UDMA (ca 40%) and Bis-GMA (ca 27%).

In our lab we have also studied by DSC the kinetics of the free radical polymerization of methyl methacrylate (MMA) using the BPO/amine initiation system [10]. N,N dimethyl-4-aminophenethyl alcohol (DMPOH) which is a newly synthesized and used amine in the preparation of acrylic dental resins and bone cements was examined and the results compared to the most commonly usedin these applications amine the DMT. For both amines the molar ratio of BPO/amine and of the reaction temperature on the polymerization kinetics was investigated. DMPOH was found to lead in slightly higher polymerization rates, lower gel times and lower molecular weights of poly(methyl methacrylate) (PMMA) than DMT. The values of these parameters for both amines were influenced by the molar ratio of BPO to amine when the product of the concentrations of these was kept constant. The highest polymerization rate occurred in the lowest gel time, resulting in polymers with the lowest molecular weight, and was observed when a molar ratio of about 1.5 BPO/amine was used. However the final monomer conversion was found to be independen of the molar ratio and amine used.

The kinetics of the free radical crosslinking polymerization of Bis-EMA and TEGDMA initiated by BPO/ DMPOH was also studied [9]. The polymerization rate vs time for several initial initiator concentrations was measured by DSC. Differences in the polymerization kinetics were observed depended on the chemical structure of dimethacrylates. Futhermore a mathematical model was developed to simulate BPO/amine initiated free radical polymerization of dimethacrylate monomers. Recently we have studied by DSC the homopolymerization and copolymerization kinetics of Bis-GMA, Bis-EMA or UDMA (base monomers) with TEGDMA (diluent) initiated by BPO/DMPOH at 37°C [11]. The maximum rate of homopolymerization of the dimethacrylates followed the order of Bis-GMA>UDMA>TEGDMA>Bis-EMA while the final degree of conversion of the corresponding homopolymers followed the order of TEGDMA>UDMA>Bis-EMA>Bis-GMA. The maximum rate of copolymerization, and the degree of conversion of copolymers changed monotonically with an increase in the TEGDMA content in the initial comonomer mixture.

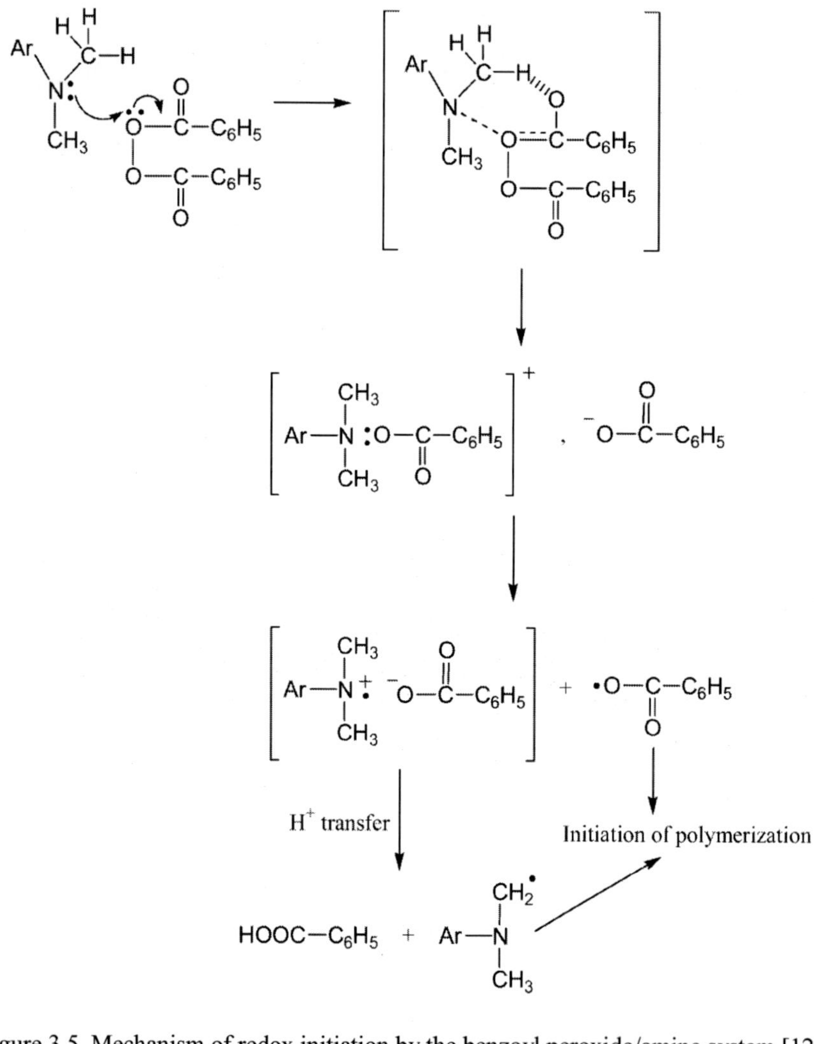

Figure 3.5. Mechanism of redox initiation by the benzoyl peroxide/amine system [12].

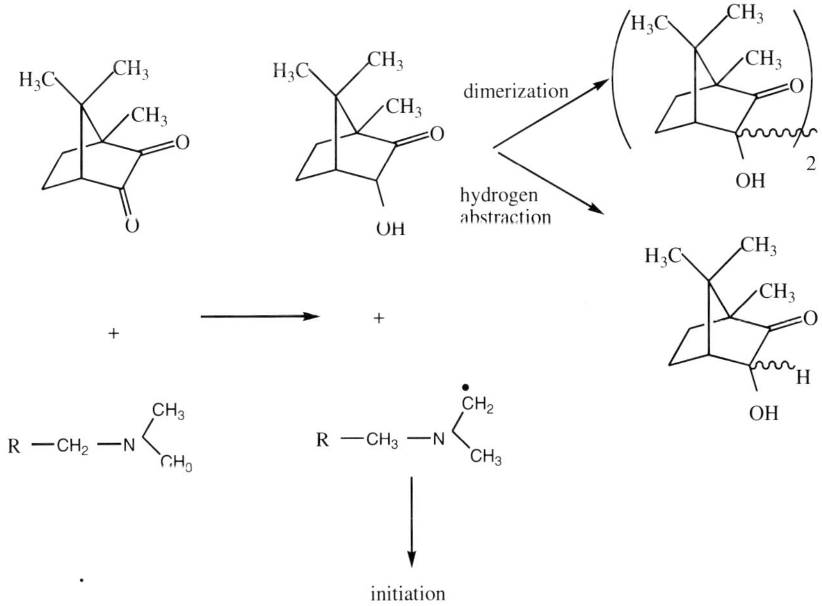

Figure 3.6. Mechanism of photoinitiation by camphorquinone/amine system.

In the above "two part" materials one of the parts incorporates the amine and the other the BPO and a stabilizer to control the start of polymerization, usually butyl hydroxytoluene (BHT). When the two parts are mixed in air at room temperature, the monomers of the mixture start to polymerize after a short time and the material starts to harden. The desired mixing time and hardening time, which is defined by the clinical application, can be adjusted by varying the content of the BPO, stabilizer and the amine. The mechanism of polymerization initiation by the BPO/DMT redox system has been used and studied for a long time. The results obtained showed that a cyclic transition molecular complex and the subsequent ion pair are formed as shown in Figure 3.5. It is accepted that both the aminoalkyl radicals and benzoyloxy radicals (RO˙) are efficient initiators for free radical polymerization.

Most of the dental composites however are light curing materials, which harden by irradiation with visible light in the wavelength range 400-500 nm. Nearly all composite manufacturers are using camphorquinone as the photoinitiator. The absorption maximum of camphorquinone is at 468 nm. Camphorquinone is a 1,2- diketone which abstract hydrogen from the co-initiator to give ketyl radicals. (Figure 3.6). Amines are the most frequently used co-initiators. The a-aminoalkyl radicals initiate the polymerization reaction while the ketyl radical mainly dimerizes or disproportionates. Light-curable dental composites combine the advantages of a long working time and fast and complete curing upon irradiation. Visible light is used in this application since UV irradiation might be harmful to the oral mucosa.

The photopolymerization is induced by irradiation with halogen lamps, emitting light in emitting light in the wavelength range of 380-500 nm. Recently new light units have been brought onto the market, such as plasma-arc lights and blue-light light-emitting diodes (LED) [13].

The free radicals prepared as described above can react then with a monomer such as vinyl monomer and initiate the polymerization process as follows:

Initiation

The free radicals can react with a monomer such as methyl methacrylate (MMA) and initiate the polymerization process as follows:

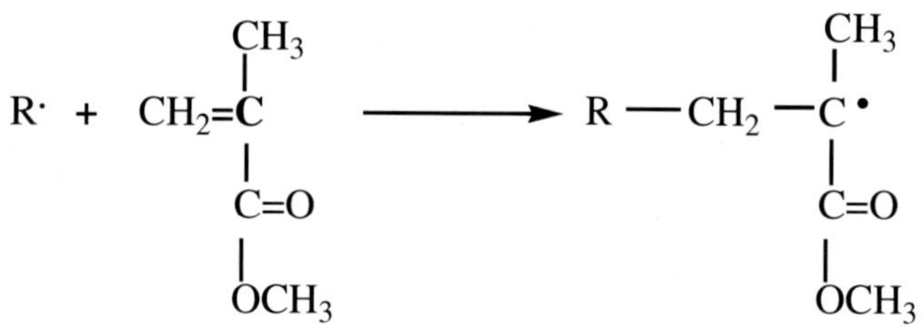

Propagation

The free radical is transferred to the monomer, which can in turn react with another monomer:

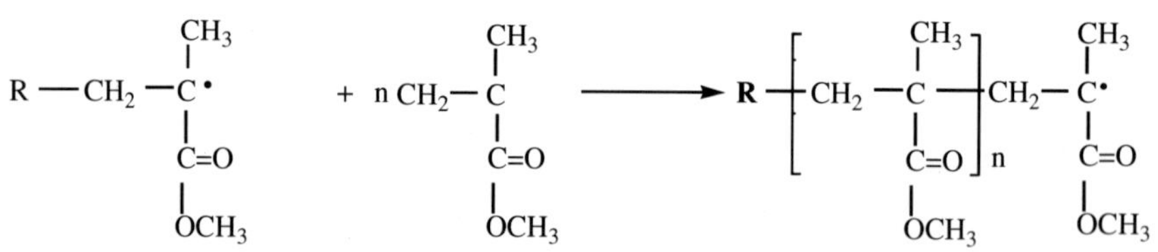

Repeating this process again and again generates the polymer chain until the growing chains collide or all of the free radicals have reacted.

Termination

Finally the free radicals can react to form a stable molecule following two ways *combination or disproportionation:*

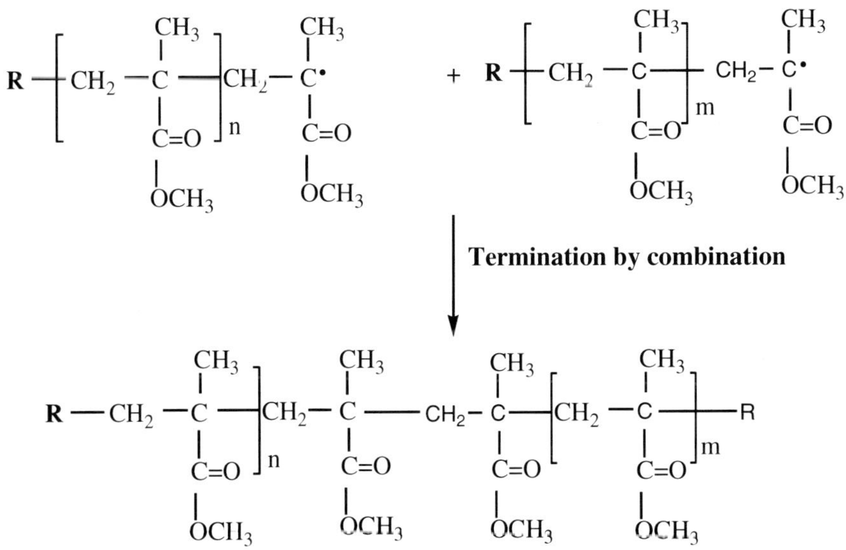

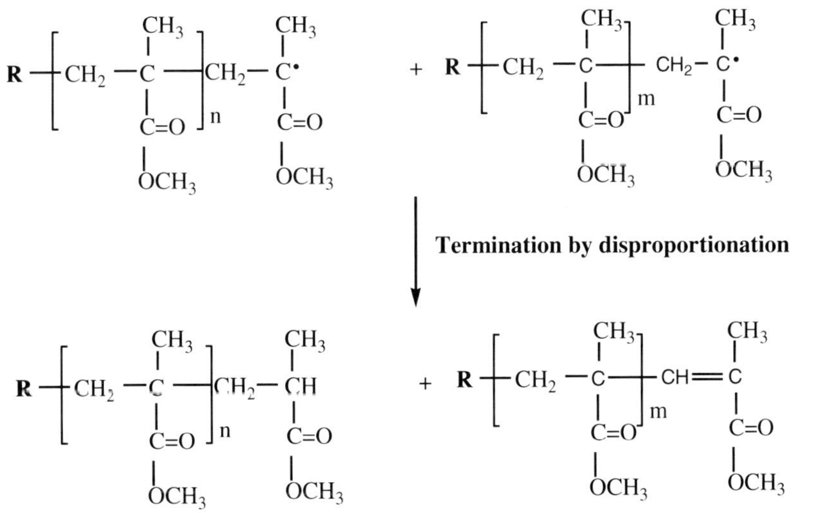

Since n and m will vary from polymeric chain to polymeric chain a wide range of long-chain molecules are produced.

The free-radical polymerization of the dimethacrylate monomers, on the contrary to MMA which gives the linear PMMA, leads to a free-dimensional network, which is shown in Figure 3.7 [14]. After the initiation of the polymerization by an initiator radical, linear propagating macroradicals are formed, because only one double bond per monomer molecule is involved at the time in the polymerization process. During the subsequent chain propagation, the macroradicals form microgel particles. At what is known as the gel point, a three dimensional (3D) polymer network is built up. The time between the initiation and the gel point is called gel time (Figure 3.8). The gel time for the polymerization of dimethacrylates is in the range of a few seconds. However to get a high double-bond conversion a longer polymerization time is needed (20-60s). After the gel point the polymerization system behaves like a visco-elastic solid. Because of the gel effect the change in density is accelerated, resulting in an increase in internal contraction stress. About 80% of the polymerization shrinkage of cross-linking dimethacrylates is responsible for the internal stress build-up that may cause the formation of a marginal gap between the resin-based filling composite and the dental hard tissue. [15].

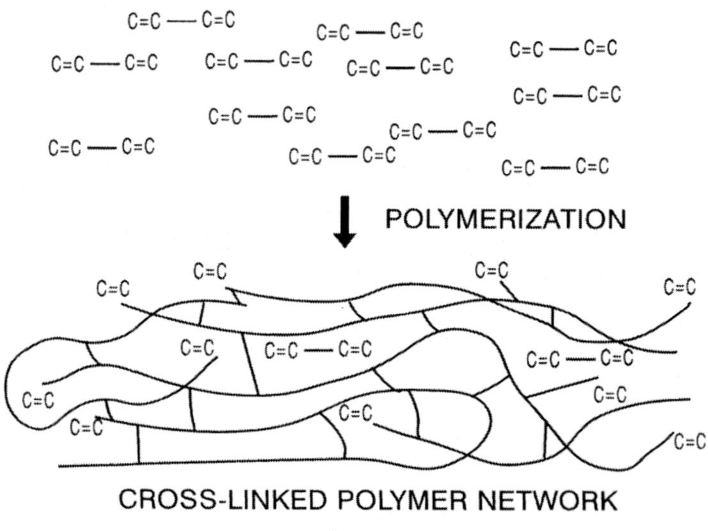

Figure 3.7. Schematic representation of the polymerization of dimethacrylate monomers to form the cross-linked polymer network of dental composites containing small amounts of unreacted monomers and many pendant methacrylate groups (C=C) [14].

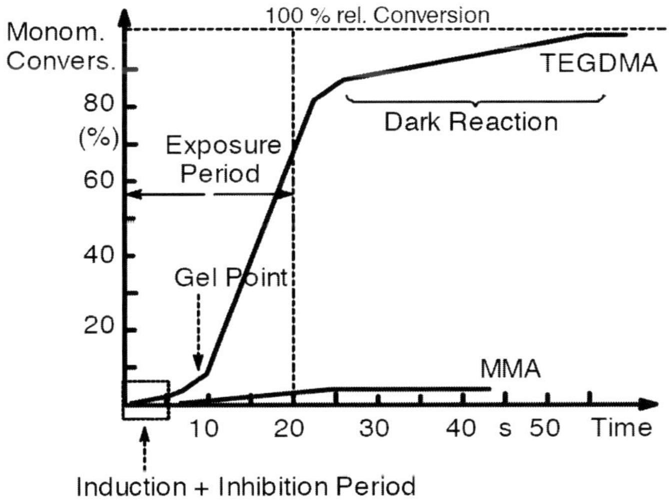

Figure 3.8. Course of cross-linking photopolymerization [16].

In general, even at a high monomer conversion, not all double bonds are consumed and radical centers are also present. The reason for this is the low flexibility of the formed polymer network at room temperature. Not all double bond radicals are available because with increasing network density, the flexibility of the polymer chains is reduced. Therefore, the residual double bond content of the formed polymer network is increasing with the functionality of the corresponding monomer. In present commercial composites, it has been verified by infrared spectrophotometry that 25-55% of the methacrylate groups remain unreacted after polymerization. An analysis of data on the extraction of unreacted species from the polymerized material suggests that less than 1 in 10 of the unreacted molecules is free and capable of being released. The result is that nearly 90% of the unreacted methacrylate groups are present on pendant molecules which have reacted at one end by linking with the polymer chain (Figure 3.7). These molecules are therefore capable of serving as internal plasticizers for the composite [14].

The selection of appropriate monomers for the formulation of a composite strongly influences the reactivity, viscosity and polymerization shrinkage of the composite paste, as well as the mechanical properties, water uptake and swelling of the cured composite. The polymerization shrinkage of the monomers used is the main disadvantage of dimethacrylates. Polymerization shrinkage compromises the adhesion of the restorative composite to the tooth structure, which may cause the formation of marginal gaps. The polymerization shrinkage of low molecular monomers is higher than that of high molecular monomers (Table 3.1). However, high molecular monomers are very viscous (Table 3.2). There is a correlation between the filler load of the composite, its polymerization shrinkage and the viscosity of the composite. Therefore, favorable special mixtures of high molecular monomers and reactive diluents in combination with different fillers are used in dental composites [6, 16].

The main deficiencies of current dental composites are polymerization shrinkage and insufficient wear resistance under high masticatory forces. Polymerization shrinkage causes a number of problems. For example polymerization shrinkage produces internal stress. Internal stress in turn produces microvoids or microcracks which impair the mechanical properties of a composite. In dental composites the most serious problem is that polymerization shrinkage impairs the adhesion to the tooth surface, which leads to the formation of marginal gaps. Therefore, a considerable number of studies have been carried out to find new ways of reducing the volume shrinkage during the polymerization of the monomer matrix. With regard to the reduction of polymerization shrinkage the application of cyclic monomers has received the most attention. It is well known that cyclic compounds possess higher densities than their linear counterparts, because they are able to arrange themselves in an orderly and close fit manner in the liquid state. In principle therefore the ring opening polymerization of cyclic monomers produces less shrinkage than the polymerization of linear monomers. In addition to the ring opening polymerization of cyclic monomers, use of preordered that is liquid crystalline cross-linkers is the second basic concept used to achieve a low-shrinkage photopolymerization system. Also hyperbranched or dendritic methacrylates and fluoride-releasing monomer systems are very promising monomers for the preparation of low-shrinking composites [2, 4, 5].

Table 3.1. Polymerization Shrinkage (ΔVp) of Dental Monomers

Monomer	ρ_{mon} (g/cm^3)	ρ_{poly} (g/cm^3)	ΔVp (%)
TEGDMA	1.072	1.250	14.3
UDMA	1.110	1.190	6.7
Bis-GMA	1.151	1.226	6.1

ρ_{mon}=density of monomer; ρ_{poly}=density of polymer.

Table 3.2. Correlation between the Molecular Weight and the Viscosity of Monomers

Monomer	Molecular Weight (g/mol)	Viscosity (mPas)
TEGDMA	286	100
UDMA	470	5,000-10,000
Bis-GMA	512	500,000-800,000

3.1.1.2. Filler

The fillers used in dental composites directly influence the radiopacity, mechanical properties such as hardness, flexural and compressive strength and thermal coefficient of expansion. The use of heavy metals such as barium and strontium incorporated in the glass provide radiopacity. Dimethacrylate monomers have a high coefficient of thermal expansion. This coefficient is reduced by the addition of fillers and ideally dental composites should have similar coefficients of thermal expansion to enamel and dentine of tooth, which is 17x10¯6/°C and about $11x10^{-6}$/ °C respectively [17]. The fillers provide the ideal means of controlling various aesthetic features such as color, translucency and fluorescence. Polymerization shrinkage largely correlates with the volumetric amount of the filler in the composite. By incorporating large amount of fillers the shrinkage is much reduced because the amount of resin used is reduced and the filler does not take part in the polymerization process. However, shrinkage is not totally eliminated and will depend on the monomers used and the amount of filler incorporated.

One of the most important considerations in the selection of filler is the optical characteristics of the composite. The monomers used in dental composites have a refractive index of approximately 1.55. Fillers with refractive indices which differ greatly from this value will cause the composite to appear optically opaque, creating an esthetic and curing problem. Because glasses can have refractive indices ranging from 1.4 to 1.9 the selection of appropriate filler for dental composites must be guided by a consideration of this important variable. The filler most used until quite recently was fused or crystalline quartz and various borosilicate or lithium aluminosilicate glasses. The glass or quartz was ground or milled into particles of various sizes ranging from approximately 0.1 μm to 100 μm. The major advantage to using quartz was that it is readily available and has an excellent optical match to the polymer matrix. However quartz has drawbacks in that it is not radiopaque and can be very abrasive to enamel. These characteristics ensured that as the surface of the composite was abraded the polymer would wear away more quickly than the fillers leaving them raised and exposed from the surface. This made the surface of the restoration rough and less enamel-like due to appreciable scattering of incident light. Thus polishability and esthetics were compromised. Most current composites are filled with radiopaque silicate particles based on oxides of barium, strontium, zinc, aluminum or zirconium [14].

The average particle size and particle size distribution of the filler is important as it determines the amount of the filler that can be added to the monomers, without the necessary handling characteristics being lost. Particle size also has a pronounced effect on the final surface finish of the composite restoration in that the smaller the filler particle size the smoother the composite will be [18].

The composites have been classified according to the type of filler employed into three main groups, the traditional or macrofilled composites, the hybrid or blended composites and the microfilled composites [5,6,14,15,18,19]. *The macrofilled composites* contain glass filler particles with a mean particle size of 10-20 nm and a largest particle size of 40 μm (Figure 3.9). These composites had the disadvantage that the surface finish was very poor with the surface having a dull appearance due to filler particles produting from the surface as the resin was preferentially removed around them. These composites are significantly less frequently used nowadays because of esthetical reasons. *The hybrid composites* contain large filler particles of an average size of 15-20 nm and also a small amount of colloidal silica which has a particle size of 0.01-0.05 μm. It should be noted that virtually all composites now contain small amounts of colloidal silica, but their behavior is very much determined by the size of the larger filler particles [18]. *Microfilled composites* containing amorphous silica were developed to address the polishing requirements of anterior restorations. These silicon dioxide particles are submicroscopic, averaging approximately 0.04 μm in diameter, though the size varies among materials. Because the filler particles in a microfilled composite are so small, they have from 1,000 to 10,000 times as much surface area as filler particles in conventional composites. The increased surface area must be wetted by the monomer matrix and which results in a significant increase in viscosity. This increase in viscosity limits the percentage filler content of the composite to approximately 35 wt%, which in turn limits the strength and stiffness of the composite. In an attempt to maximize filler loading while minimizing increase in viscosity, a two-stage procedure for the incorporation of the filler has been developed. A very high filler loaded material is first produced by one of a variety of techniques. This material is then polymerized and ground into particles of 10-40 μm in size, which is subsequently used as filler for more resin. This process effectively maximizes percentage filler content to about 50-60 wt% (35-45 vol%). The small size of the particles allowed these composites to be polished without preferential abrasion, thus producing smooth surfaces and excellent esthetics. The wink link in microfilled composites is the bond between the prepolymerized filler and the organic matrix. The resin fillers are heat cured and do not form covalent chemical bonds with the polymerizing matrix due to the lack of available methacrylate groups on their surface. Therefore, they become debonded and dislodged under high stresses.

Within the last few years several new types of polymer composites have been introduced to the market. Whether these products actually constitute a new type of material is debatable, however they are being marketed and classified as such, so it is important to be aware of them. The new classes are packable or condensable composites, universal composites, reinforced microfills and nanofilled composites. A number of problems have been associated with using polymer composites for posterior restorations including staining, marginal ditching, post operative sensitivity, increased wear compared to metallic restorations and difficulties in obtaining adequate interproximal contacts. In an effort to overcome these problems new composites called *packable or condensable composites* are being promoted as amalgam alternatives and not substitutes. The preferred term for these polymer composites is "packable" rather "condensable", because during placement they are simply being packed rather than condensed. The compositions and physical reported by manufacturers reveal that none of the materials represents a remarkable improvement over the properties of more traditional universal composites. The distinguishing characteristics of all packable compositions are less stickiness or stiffer viscosity than conventional composites, which allow them to be placed in a manner that somewhat resembles amalgam placement. Packable composites may be selected as alternatives to amalgam or conventional universal composites, but they are not equal to or better than dental amalgam in all respects. Also, in most cases, mechanical properties of packable composites are not substantially better than those of most conventional universal composites.

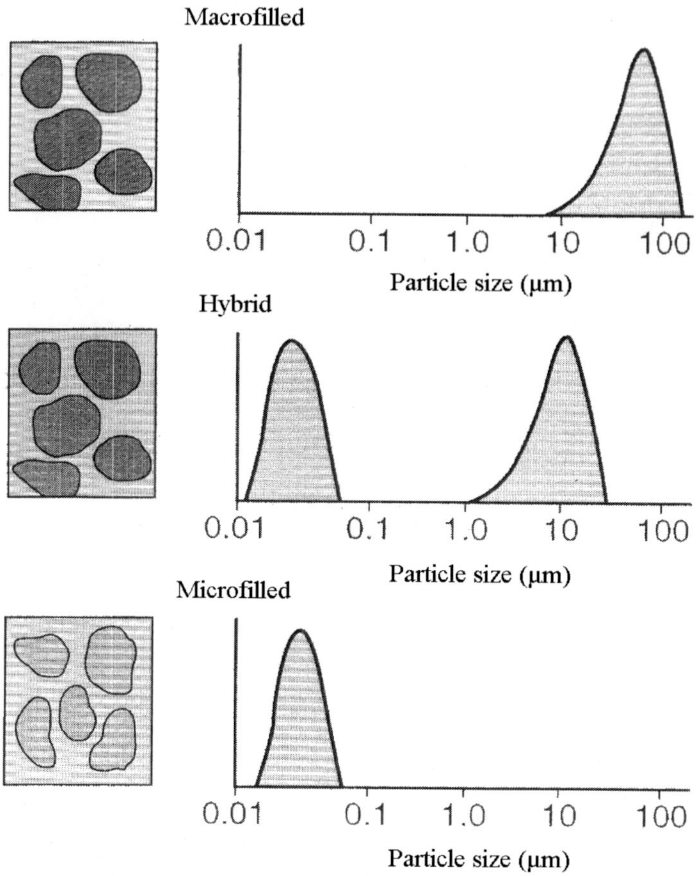

Figure 3.9. A classification of composites based on filler type with the horizontal axis as the logarithmic scale of the particle size.

Universal polymer composites are purported by their manufacturers to have the physical and mechanical of a hybrid along with the esthetics and polishability of a microfill. As such their manufacturers claim they obviate a clinician's need for a separate hybrid and microfill. *Reinforced microfills* have been introduced in the market perhaps in an attempt to compete with the universal polymer composites. These composites generally have higher percentage filler content than traditional microfills and because of this it is claimed that they are appropriate for posterior as well as anterior use.

Nanofilled polymer composites are different from other types of composites in that they contain nanofillers. Nanotechnology has led to the development of a new polymer composite characterized by containing nanoparticles measuring approximately 25 nm and nanoaggregates of approximately 75 nm, which are made up of zirconium/silica or nanosilica particles. The aggregates are treated with silane so that they bind to the polymer matrix. The distribution of the filler (aggregates and nanoparticles) gives a high load up to 79.5% [20]. As the particle size is smaller composites made with this type of particle give the restoration a better finish, which is observed in its surface texture and the likelihood of the material's biodegrading over time is reduced. This technology has also achieved sufficiently competent mechanical properties for the composite to be indicated for use in the anterior and posterior sectors. It should also be mentioned that the lower size of the particles leads to less curing shrinkage, creates less cusp wall deflection and reduces the presence of microfissures in the enamel edges, which are responsible for marginal leakage, color changes, bacterial penetration and possible post-operative sensitivity. The drawback is that since the particles are so small they do not reflect light, so they are combined with larger-sized particles with an average diameter within visible light wavelengths (i.e. around or below 1μm) to improve their optical performance and act as a substrate [21].

3.1.1.3. Coupling Agent

During the initial development of dental composites it was shown that the acquisition of good properties in the composite was dependent upon the formation of a strong bond between the inorganic filler particles and the organic polymer matrix. If there is a breakdown of this interface, the stresses developed under load will not be effectively distributed throughout the composite. The interface will act as a primary source for fracture, leading to the subsequent disintegration of the composite. In most mineral reinforced dental composites the primary interphasial linkage between the polymer matrix and the filler phase is by chemical bond formation mediated by a dual functional organosilane, termed a silane coupling agent [22-25]. In dental composites based on dimethacrylates adhesion between the polymeric matrix and the reinforcing filler is usually achieved by use of the silane coupling agent 3-methacryloxypropyltrimethoxysilane (γ-MPS), a bifunctional molecule capable of reacting via its alkoxysilane groups with the filler and itself and with the polymer matrix by virtue of its methacrylate functional group (Figure 3.10).

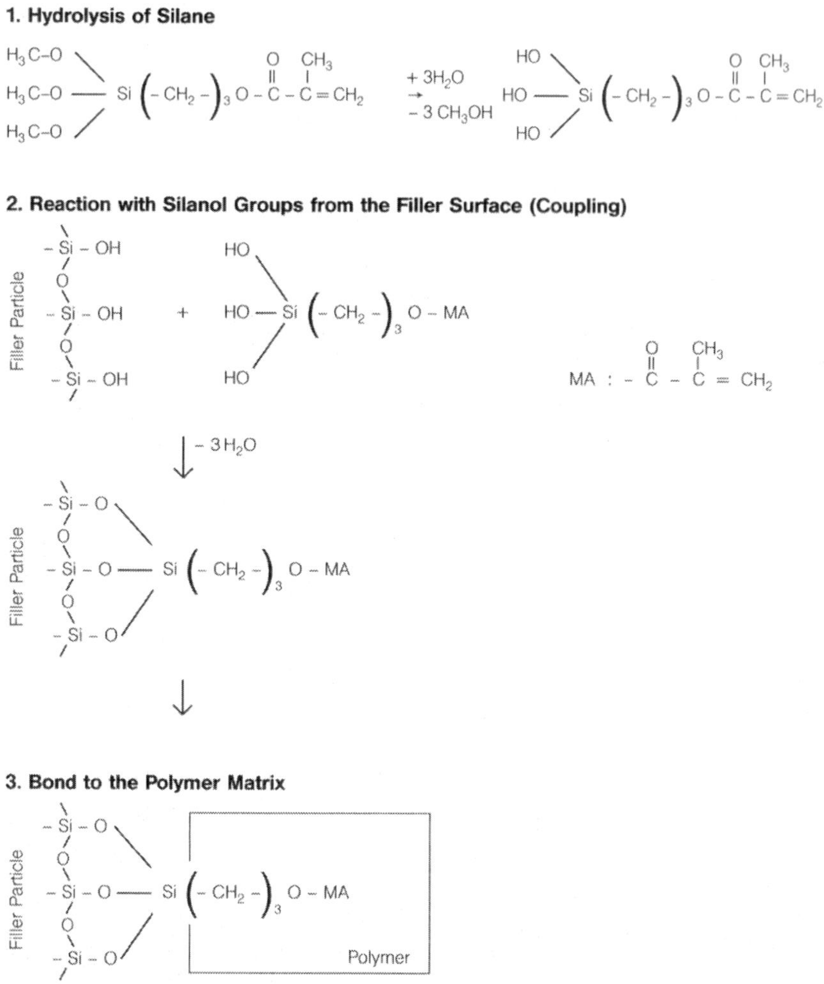

Figure 3.10. Schematic representation of the silane treatment and filler-matrix bond.

The particulate glass fillers are usually presilanized by deposition from dilute aqueous/organic solutions of γ-MPS. Bulk deposition of the silane by spray-on techniques during mechanical mixing or grinding of the fillers is also employed. The treated fillers are then incorporated by mechanical mixing into a mixture of dimethacrylates which contained an initiator for subsequent light-curing of the resulting composite. The silanization procedure used to coat the filler particles is an important factor in determining the extent of coverage of the fillers. When applied from solvents, the type of solvent, the amount of water, pH, catalyst and temperature used are all important factors in determining the type of a broad more gradient-like transition zone (interphase) that forms between the continuous or polymer matrix phase and the dispersed phase [26,27]. The *in situ* silanization of glass fillers, also referred as integral blending, is simpler than presilanization and involves simply adding the γ-MPS as a comonomer to the dimethacrylate monomer mixture and then forming a composite paste by admixture with unsilanized glass filler [28].

In our recent work silanization of Aerosil OX50 was performed by mixing a certain amount of γ-MPS in cyclohexane in the presence of 2% by volume of n-propylamine used as catalyst [25]. The use of n-propylamine accelerates the silanization of the silica and yields the most stable interfacial silicon-silane bonds. [27]. The silanized silica was dried at 95°C for 1h and at 80 °C for 20h. This silanization procedure was followed by Antonucci et al. in their attempt to study the interphase effects in dental nanocomposites [29-31]. The silane layer orientation that develops (parallel or perpendicular to the silica surface) is dependent on the silane concentration and is an important parameter that determinates many of the physicochemical and mechanical properties of the interphase and in turn those of the composite. This orientation can be determinate by FT-IR spectroscopy [32, 33]. The FT-IR spectra of Aerosil OX50 treated with various amount of γ-MPS in our work [25] are shown in Figure 3.11. The band at 1638 cm^{-1} is the stretching vibration of the C=C bond in γ-MPS and the bands at 1722 and 1706 cm^{-1} are C=O modes. The band at 1722 cm^{-1} is due to the free carbonyl (C=O) stretching vibration and the peak at 1706 cm^{-1} is characteristic of the carbonyl groups which form hydrogen bonds with the silica or adjacent silane hydroxyls. There is a single carbonyl stretching frequency at 1706 cm^{-1} for amounts 1 wt% and 2.5 wt% and overlapped bands at 1722 and 1706 cm^{-1} for amounts 5%, 7.5% and 10 wt%. As the amount of γ-MPS increased the intensity of the 1722 cm^{-1} peak continued to increase. The ratio of intensities of peaks A_{1706} / A_{1722} takes values 1.06, 1.10 and 1.21 for the amounts correspondingly 5%, 7.5% and 10 wt%. The carbonyl vibration of neat unhydrolyzed γ-MPS absorbs at 1720 cm^{1}.

The observed shift to lower frequency when γ-MPS is absorbed on silica is caused by hydrogen bonding of the carbonyl group with the hydroxyls of silica and can be used to characterize parallel monomolecular coverage on silica surface [32,34]. This interaction is spectroscopically identified by a single band at 1706 cm^{-1} (Figure 3.11). In Figure 3.11 the hydrogen bonded structure is observed exclusively up to a surface concentration of 2.5 wt% and therefore this concentration defines parallel monomolecular coverage on silica.

This finding is in agreement with that reported by Jang and Kim [35]. Illustrative representation of the experimentally observed parallel monomolecular structure on the silica is shown in Figure 3.12. The carbonyl functionality has hydrogen bonding interaction with surface silanols and the hydrolyzed trialkoxy also has covalent surface linkages. Since both ends of the molecule have surface interactive functionalities, the molecule must have a parallel orientation relative to the surface (Figure 3.12a).

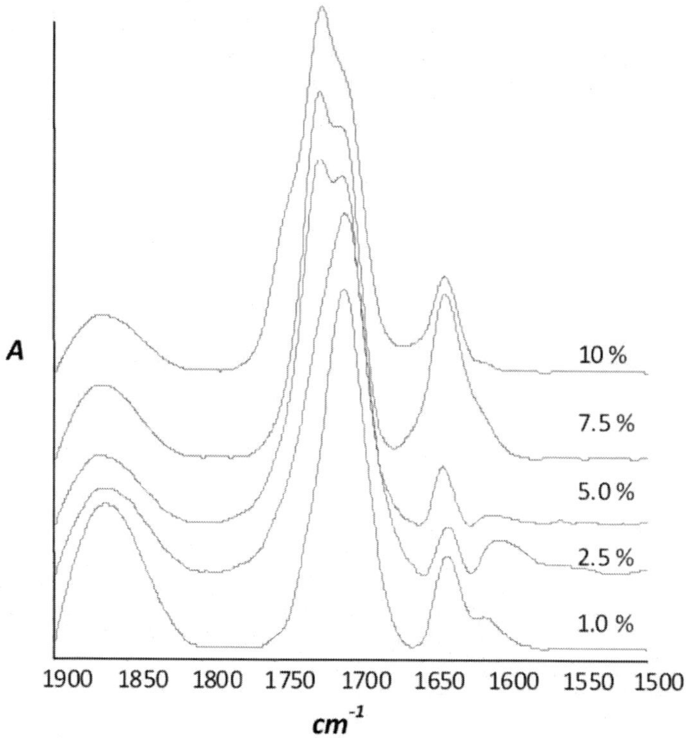

Figure 3.11. FT-IR spectra of silane treated silica surface with increasing amounts of silane γ-MPS (in wt%): 1.0, 2.5, 5.0, 7.5, 10.0 [25].

FT-IR spectroscopic characterization of parallel monomolecular coverage can also be used to calculate the area occupied per silane molecule on the silica surface. Aerosil OX50 has a specific surface area of 50 m^2/g. Parallel monomolecular coverage was spectroscopically identified at a concentration of 2.5 wt% or 2.5 mg/g or $6.064x10^{19}$ molecules/g. In conjunction with the specific surface area of Aerosil OX 50 molecular coverage is calculated to be

$1.2x10^{18}$ molecules/m^2. When this value is converted to surface area per molecule the γ-MPS molecule occupies 0.83 nm^2. It is worth noting that Miller and Ishida [29] studied the monomolecular coverage by γ-MPS of clay and lead oxide particles found that the surface area occupied by each γ-MPS molecule is 0.60 and 0.59 nm^2 respectively. This value compares closely with an area of 0.55 nm^2 per molecule calculated from the space filling projection of the molecule interacting with the surface through its silanol and carbonyl functionalities [33]. Also Söderholm and Shang [32] found that each γ-MPS molecule occupies at least 1.11 nm^2 of colloidal silica, while Nishiyama et al. [36] found that each γ-MPS molecule occupies 0.5-0.67 nm^2 of colloidal silica.

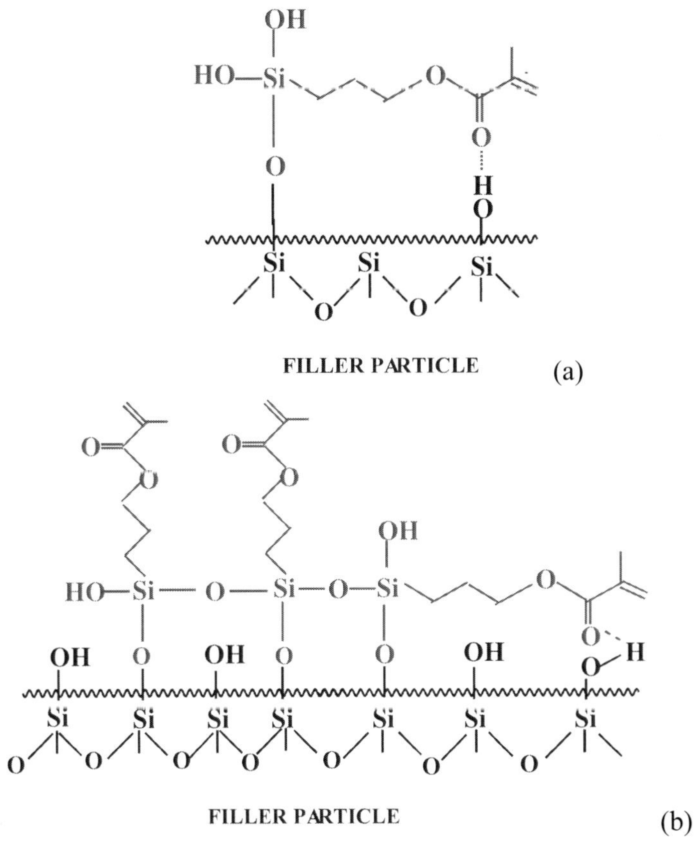

Figure 3.12. Simplified illustrative molecular structure of (a) parallel and (b) random monomolecular γ-MPS molecules.

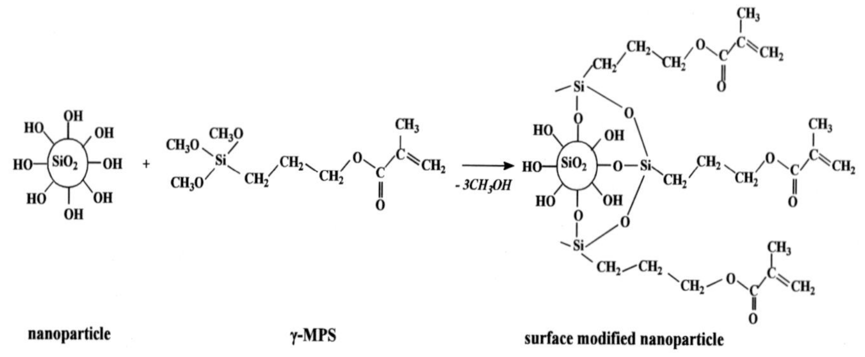

Figure 3.13. Idealized picture of γ-MPS surface grafted silica particle, when silane amounts higher than 2.5 wt% are used.

At higher silane amounts (>2.5 wt%) silane molecules form a layer around the filler particles which must have according to the FTIR spectra of the corresponding silanized silicas random (parallel and perpendicular) orientation relative to the silica surface [37, 38] (Figure 3.12b). Idealized picture of γ-MPS surface grafted silica particle (perpendicular orientation) when silane amounts higher than 2.5 wt% are used is showed in Figure 3.13. Silane molecules oriented perpendicularly to the filler surface area occupy less filler surface area (0.24 nm^2 per molecule) [33] making it possible to increase the number of silane molecules that can react with the filler surface. Thus differences in molecular orientations are likely to have a significant impact on the filler-matrix bond strength of dental composites.

Another way to approach the problem of orientation of silane layer on silica surface is to assume that the silane molecules bond to the silica surface only via the OH-groups available on that surface. In Aerosil OX50 surface silanol groups exist in both an isolated state and bridged by hydrogen bonds. The total number of silanol groups was found to be 2.1 OH-groups/nm^2 from which 1.8 OH-groups/nm^2 are isolated [39]. If we assume that all 2.1 OH-groups react with one γ-MPS molecule each, then 0.0433 g of γ-MPS per 1 g of Aerosil OX 50 is needed. Instead assume that each isolated OH-group reacts with one molecule of γ-MPS. With this assumption 0.0371 g of γ-MPS must be used to consume each isolated OH-group per gram of Aerosil OX 50 that was used. In this study the FTIR spectroscopy showed that the critical γ-MPS concentration needed for complete surface reaction is 2.5 wt% which corresponds to 0.025 g of γ-MPS per g of silica. This result shows that only the isolated OH-groups react with the silane molecules and most probably two isolated OH-groups may react with a silanol and the carbonyl group of each silane molecule. This finding is in line with that reported by Söderholm and Shang [32] for silanization of colloidal silica with different amount of γ-MPS.

The amount of γ-MPS attached to Aerosil OX 50 surface was quantitatively determined by thermogravimetric analysis (TGA) and is presented in Table 3.3. TGA of the samples showed one-step weight loss that occurred between 270-500 °C in nitrogen and between 260-470 °C in air, indicating that only chemically bound silane molecules remained on the surface of the silica, since the physically adsorbed silane is removed at lower temperatures (50-150 °C) [40] and no such a weight loss was observed in our TGA curves at that temperature range. The drying process which we applied during the preparation of silanized silica, 1 h at 95 °C and 20 h at 80 °C under vacuum, seems to remove the physically adsorbed silane simply by evaporation. TGA data from Table 3.3 show that for silica silanated in solution of γ-MPS 2.5 wt-%, which is the maximum concentration for a parallel orientation of silane molecules on silica surface (a single band at 1706 cm^{-1} in FTIR spectra, Fig. 3.11) the number of γ-MPS/nm^2 is 1.10. This value corresponds to 0.91 nm^2 per γ-MPS molecule. When higher amounts of silane were used the number of γ-MPS/nm^2 is 1.90-2.22 which corresponds to 0.53-0.45 nm^2 per γ-MPS molecule. TGA curves showed also a small weight loss at approximately 500°C which is due to condensation of surface silanols [40].

Study of the mechanical properties of composites prepared with the use of various amounts of silane γ-MPS showed that no significant statistic difference exists between the flexural strength and flexural modulus values of composites with different silane contents. Dynamic elastic modulus E' showed a maximum value for the composite contained 5 wt% silane. The composites with the higher amounts of silane showed the lower values for tanδ at the T_g revealing that these composites have better interfacial adhesion between filler and matrix [25].

Generally the efficacy of a silane coupling agent is determined by the overall degrees of reaction of the silane with the glass filler (oxane bond formation) with itself (by siloxane formation) and with the polymer matrix (by graft copolymerization). The oxane bond (silicon-oxygen-silicon) that forms between the silane agent and the mineral filler can be especially vulnerable to hydrolysis, because this covalent bond has significant ionic character [23, 27]. By contrast, the carbon-carbon covalent bond that forms between the silane and the polymer matrix is considerable more stable to hydrolytic attack than the silicon-oxygen covalent bond. For a given polymer/filler system, the physical-chemical nature of the silane agent, (e.g. chemical structure, molecular size, degree of hydrophobicity, reactivity, functionality), the silanization procedure employed, the silane layer orientation that develops and the extent of filler coverage are important parameters that determine many of the physicochemical and mechanical properties of the interphase, and in turn, those of composite. The durability of the interface/interphase in the oral environment and its ability to transfer stresses between the polymer and filler phases during mastication are especially important properties for dental composites to have [23].

One approach aimed at improving the quality and durability of the filler/matrix interface involves the use of more hydrophobic and flexible silane coupling agents than γ-MPS such as the 10-(methacryloyloxy)-decyltrimethoxysilane (MDTMS) [41-43]. The decrease in the flexural strength upon storage of the composite sample in water can be reduced by surface modification with the more hydrophobic silane MDTMS. But the overall mechanical properties achieved with this silane bearing the flexible decyl spacer are worse than those attained with the silane possessing the propyl spacer. A further advantage of using fillers silanized with MDTMS is that this surface treatment enables higher loadings to be achieved [44].

Table 3.3. Amount of silane γ-MPS attached on the silica Aerosil OX50 surface determined by TGA of silanizated silica in nitrogen or air atmosphere

Amount of γ-MPS used in silanization (wt %)	TGA weight loss (%)	Silane attached on the silica surface		
		wt-%	μmol / m^2	molecules / nm^2
From TGA in nitrogen				
1.0	0.49	0.96	0.77	0.46
2.5	1.16	2.27	1.83	1.10
5.0	2.00	3.91	3.15	1.90
7.5	2.21	4.32	3.48	2.09
10	2.34	4.57	3.68	2.22
From TGA in air				
1.0	0.50	0.98	0.79	0.47
2.5	1.17	2.29	1.84	1.11
5.0	2.14	4.18	3.37	2.03
7.5	2.32	4.53	3.65	2.20
10	2.43	4.75	3.82	2.30

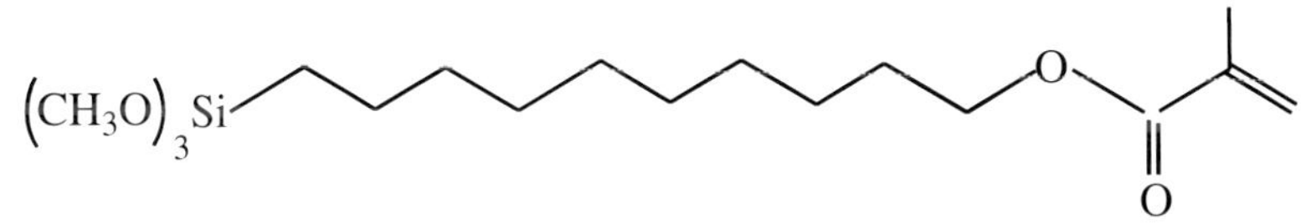

MDTMS

In addition to altering the chemical structure of silane coupling agents through varying the length and structure of the segment R between the methacrylate moiety and the alkoxysilicon group, structural variations also can be made in the number of methacrylate and alkoxysilicon groups. Such a multifunctional silane agent was prepared from the reaction of Bis-GMA and 3-isocyanatopropyltriethoxysilane and is shown in Figure 3.14. This multifunctional type of silane agent conferred enhanced hydrolytic durability on glass-filled composites when compared with similar composites filled with glass treated with γ-MPS only, presumably because of the increased degree of crosslinking in the interphase [45].

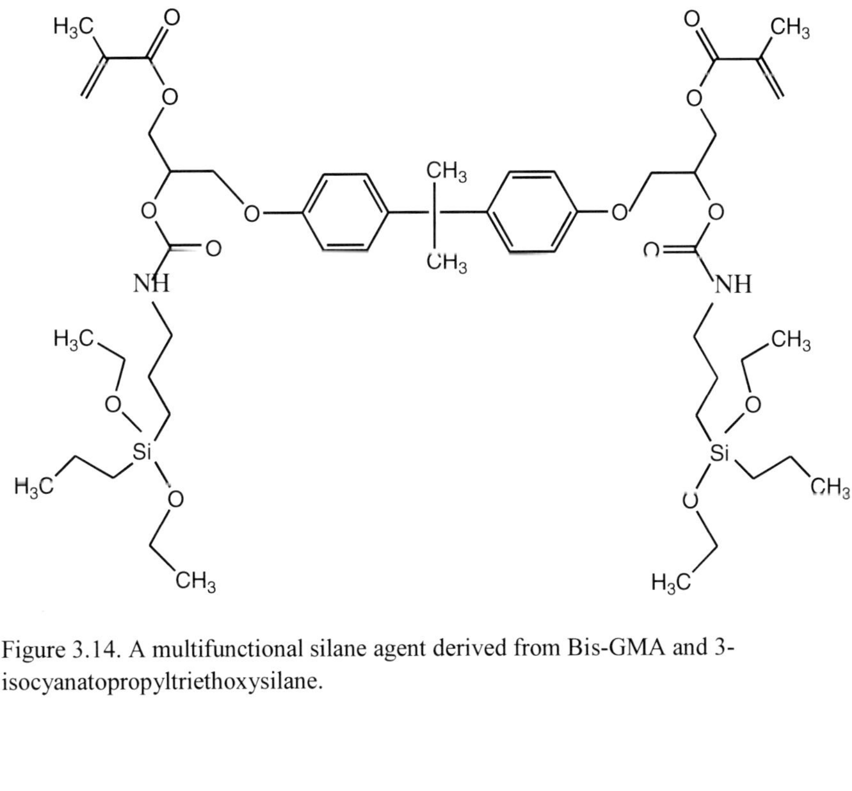

Figure 3.14. A multifunctional silane agent derived from Bis-GMA and 3-isocyanatopropyltriethoxysilane.

Another silane which shows promising results is the adduct of glycerol dimethacrylate and 3-(isocyanato)propyltriethoxysilane (UDMS) which has crosslinking properties. Less brittleness of the cured composites is observed after storage in water. Furthermore, the mechanical properties are better than those achieved with MDTMS [46].

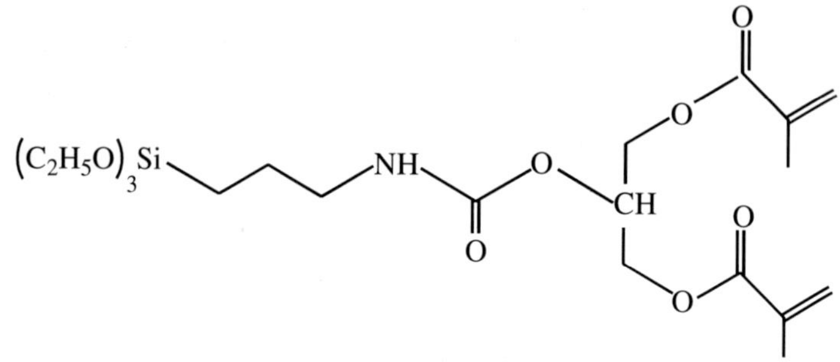

UDMS

Plueddmann and Pape found that many composites are stronger and resist water better when an appropriate silane mixture, rather than a single silane is used. Mixtures of phenyltrimethoxysilane with aminofunctional silanes have been used and showed improved water resistance and thermal stability [26,47]. Kurata and Yamazaki [48] and Craig and Dootz [49] also showed that fluorinated hydrophobic silanes increase the hydrolytic stability of the interface between filler and polymer matrix, even though they do not contain C=C bonds capable of reacting with the monomer matrix. Nihei et all used a mixture of γ-MPS with one of the following hydrophobic fluoroalkyltrimethoxysilanes [50]:

CF_3 - $(CH_2)_2$-$Si(OCH_3)_3$	trifluoropropyl-trimethoxysilane
C_4F_9 - $(CH_2)_2$-$Si(OCH_3)_3$	nonafluorohexyl- trimethoxysilane
C_6F_{13} - $(CH_2)_2$-$Si(OCH_3)_3$	tridecafluorooctyl- trimethoxysilane
C_8F_{17} - $(CH_2)_2$-$Si(OCH_3)_3$	heptadecafluorodecyl- trimethoxysilane
$C_{10}F_{21}$- $(CH_2)_2$-$Si(OCH_3)_3$	henicosafluorododecyl- trimethoxysilane

Recently Matinlinna et al. evaluated a novel silane system consisting of a functional silane + a non-functional crosslinking silane and found that silane blends might enhance the adhesion significantly *in vitro* [51,52].The functional silanes used are the γ-MPS, the 3-acryloyloxy-propyltrimethoxysilane, N-[3-(trimetoxysilyl)propyl]ethylenediamine or [3-

(triethoxysilyl)propyl]urea and the non-functional crosslinking silane is the 2-bis-(triethoxysilyl)ethane (Figure 3.15). Some less studied organofunctional silanes such as 3-(3-methoxy-4-methacryloyloxyphenyl)propyltrimethoxy silane [53] and reactive organosilanes, such as 3-isocyanatopropyltriethoxysilane [54] demonstrate a significant improvement in the adhesion promotion in vitro (Figure 3.16).

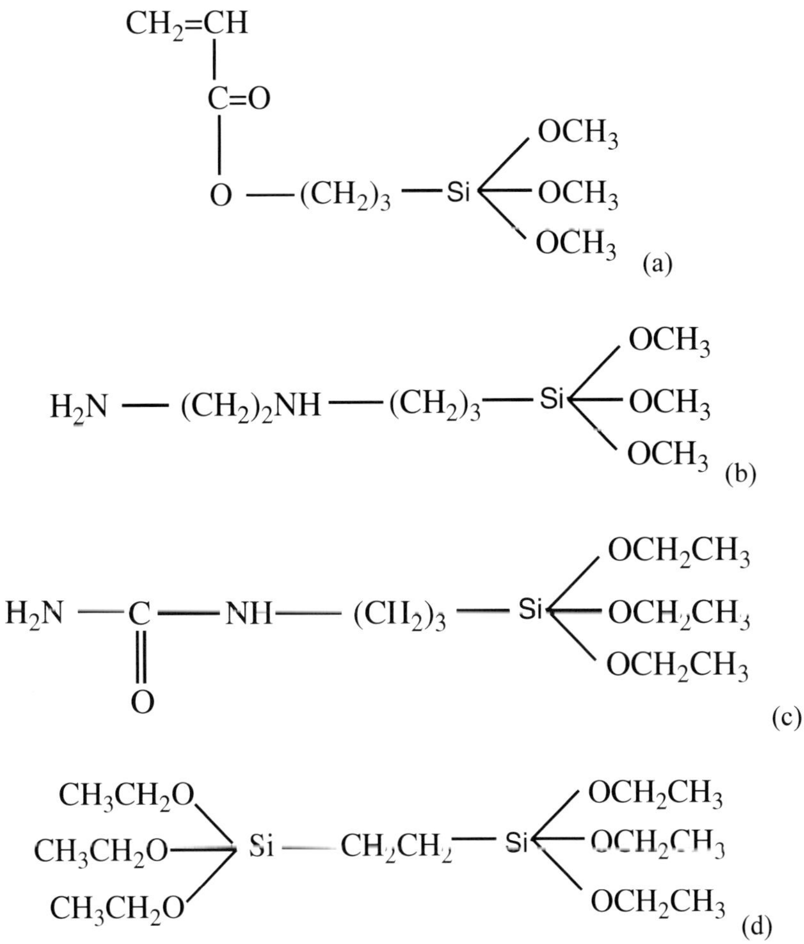

Figure 3.15. Functional silanes: (a) 3-acryloyloxypropyltrimethoxysilane, (b) N-[3-(trimetoxysilyl)propyl]ethylenediamine, (c) [3-(triethoxysilyl)propyl]urea. A non-functional crosslinking silane: (d) 2-bis-(triethoxysilyl)ethane.

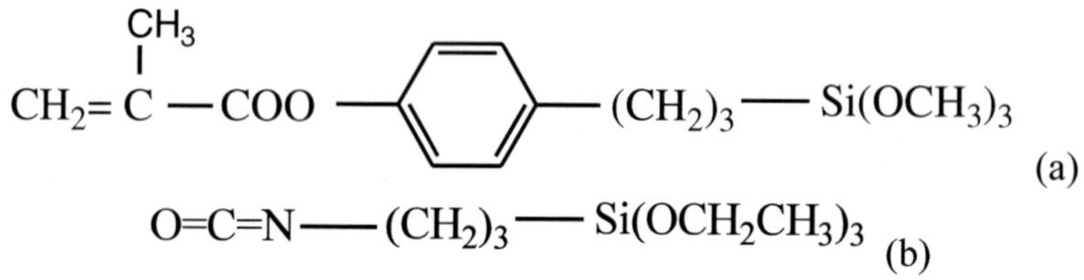

Figure 3.16. (a) 3-(3-methoxy-4-methacryloyloxyphenyl)propyltrimethoxy silane. (b) 3-isocyanatopropyltriethoxysilane.

Antonucci and al. suggest recently the dual silanization of silica nanoparticles with blends of reactive γ-MPS and non-reactive n-octyltrimethoxy silane (OMTS). OTMS does not react with the polymer matrix, but interacts mainly through weak van der Waals forces. This dual silanization offers a number of potential advantages compared to silanization with γ-MPS only. These advantages include improved uncured paste handling characteristics, higher double bond conversion during light-curing of composite, improved durability in the aqueous oral environment and lower polymerization stress [29-31].

In our lab we have studied recently the sorption characteristics of water or ethanol/water solution (75 vol% / 25 vol%) by dental nanocomposites consisted of a Bis-GMA/TEGDMA (50/50wt/wt) matrix and silica nanoparticles (Aerosil OX50) as filler, silanized with various silanes. The silanes used were 3-[(1,3(2)-dimethacryloyloxypropyl)-2(3)-oxycarbonylamido] propyltriethoxysilane, which is a urethane dimethacrylate silane (UDMS), 3-methacryloxypropyltrimethoxysilane (γ-MPS), octyltrimethoxysilane (OTMS), blends UDMS/OTMS (50/50 wt/wt) or blends γ-MPS/OTMS (50/50 wt/wt). Silane structrure used for the silanization of nanosilica was found to affect the sorption behavior of water or ethanol/water solution (37 °C) by the composites. The composite containing the UDMS with the hydrophilic urethane group showed the highest sorbed amount of water. The composite with the OTMS, which does not contain a methacrylate moiety and cannot react with the dimethacrylate monomers, showed the highest solubility both in water and ethanol/water. In all composites the amount of sorbed ethanol/water solution is much higher than that of water. OTMS-composite sorbed the highest amount of ethanol/water and the γ-MPS-composite with the 3-methacryloxypropyltrimethoxysilane (γ-MPS) the lowest [55].

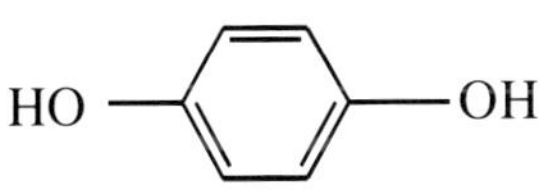

(A)

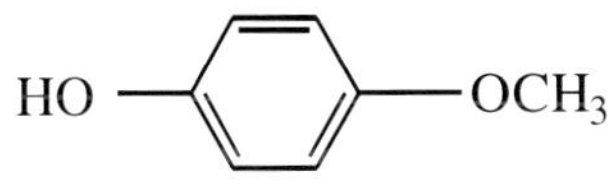

(B)

Figure 3.17. (A) Hydroquinone (1,4-dihydroxybenzene); (B) Monomethyl ether of hydroquinone.

Also we have studied the dynamic mechanical properties of the above mentioned nanocomposites i.e. the storage modulus (E'), loss modulus (E''), tangent delta (tan δ), and glass transition temperature (Tg). Measurements were performed in samples immediately after curing and samples stored in water at 37°C for 1, 7, 30, or 120 days. OTMS-composite in which OTMS does not form covalent bond with the dimethacrylate matrix showed lower elastic modulus both in dry and wet conditions. The ability of bifunctional UDMS for crosslinking was found not to increase the elastic behavior of the composite, as it was expected, compared with that of γ-MPS-composite, because of the high amount of the silane used. After immersion in water the elastic modulus of OTMS-composite remained constant, while that of the other composites increased after 1 day and then remained constant up to 120 days. [56].

3.1.1.4. Polymerization Inhibitor

Since dimethacrylate monomers will polymerize on storage, an inhibitor is necessary. Hydroquinone has been widely used, but was responsible for causing discoloration of the material. The monomethyl ether of hydroquinone is now used (Figure 3.17). Only a few parts per million of this compound are required [57].

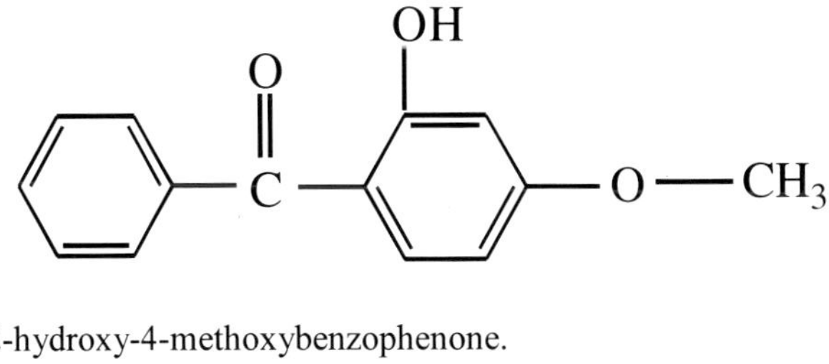

Figure 3.18. 2-hydroxy-4-methoxybenzophenone.

3.1.1.5. Ultra Violet Stabilizer

To prevent discoloration of composites in service compounds are incorporated which absorb electromagnetic radiation. Clinical evidence suggests that this improves color stability (example 2-hydroxy-4-methoxybenzophenone, Figure 3.18.) [57].

3.1.1.6. Pigment

Inorganic are also added in small amounts to provide shades that match the majority of tooth shades. Typically composites are provided in 10 or more shades covering the normal range of human teeth (yellow to gray). Highly pigmented tins can be mixed with the standard shades to match the color of teeth outside the normal range. Special shades for incisal edges of anterior restorations and for bleached teeth are also available.

3.1.2. Properties of Polymeric Dental Composites

Important properties of polymeric dental composites are: (1) polymerization shrinkage (2) water sorption and solubility (3) thermal properties (4) radiopacity (5) color (6) biocompatibility (7) fluoride release and (8) mechanical properties (9) dynamic mechanical properties (10) wear and (11) hardness.

3.1.2.1. Polymerization Shrinkage

The polymerization shrinkage of a composite is depended upon the chemical structure and the amount of monomers used for the preparation of polymer matrix. Most dental composites use monomers with comparable polymerization shrinkage values. Ideally the polymerization shrinkage of the composite should be as low as possible as this enhances marginal adaptation, reduces the possibility of breakdown of the bond to the tooth tissues and inhibits the development of recurrent caries. The traditional amalgam minimizes this problem because they show a slight expansion on setting and in due course the gap fills with corrosion products. The lower limit of polymerization shrinkage shown by current dental composites is around 2.0 vol%. Even with acid etching of enamel and dentin and use of bonding agents polymerization shrinkage has been implicated as a primary source of interfacial breakdown, resulting in visible white lines or invisible cracks in the enamel and polymer matrix at the margins. The latter are only visible clinically when using transillumination and magnification. During the setting process shrinkage stresses develop because the material is constrained by the adhesion to the cavity walls. These stresses can be sufficient to cause breakdown of the interfacial bond, whereby the advantage of the adhesive procedure is lost. This is particularly so for the bond to dentine, which is less strong than that achieved to acid-etched enamel and as a consequence the shrinkage tends to occur towards the acid-etched enamel-bonded interface if the bond to the dentine breaks down (Figure 3.19). The gap that forms between the restoration and the dentine will give rise to postoperative sensitivity due to the hydrodynamic effect. If any of the margins are in dentine then the breakdown of the bond will also give rise to marginal leakage. This is especially a problem when composites are placed subgingivally in proximal boxes [18].

Two techniques have been proposed to overcome or minimize the effect of polymerization shrinkage. One method is to insert and polymerize the composite in layers, thus reducing the effective shrinkage. The second method is to prepare a laboratory (indirect) composite inlay on a die and then to cement the inlay to the tooth with a thin layer of low viscosity composite cement [58].

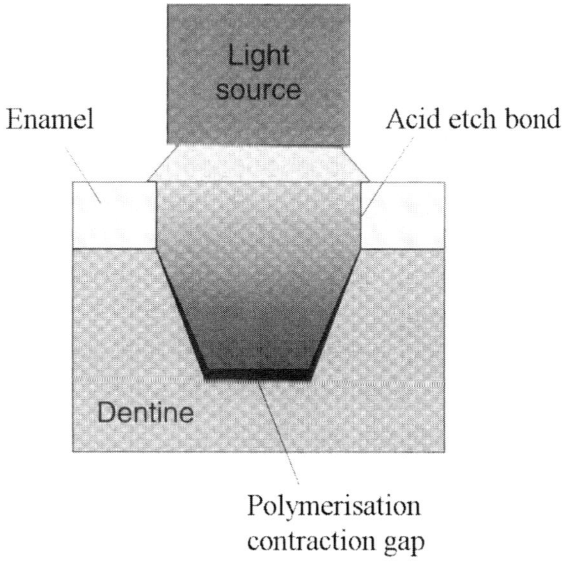

Figure 3.19. Gap formation as a consequence of polymerization shrinkage [18].

In our recent work [59] the volumetric shrinkage of two current light-cured polymer composites was measured based on the Arcimedes Principle. The densities of uncured composites were first measured, using an analytical balance. From each test material uncured sphere-shaped specimens, were carefully formed in such a way that trapped air bubbles were avoided. Since the uncured materials were rather sticky, a thin polyester film (thickness 0.05) was fixed on the special holder of the balance and its mass was measured in air and in water. Next, the respective material sample was carefully placed on the polyester film and the mass of the whole assembly was measured again in air and in water. Slight deformations of the material during the test were of no importance since they do not influence the density. The mass of each material was calculated by subtracting the mass of the polyester film from the mass of the whole assembly. Now the density of the uncured material (ρ_{uncured}) was computed. The volumetric shrinkage (ΔV) was calculated using the following equation:

$$\Delta V\% = 100x(1 - \frac{\rho_{uncured}}{\rho_{cured}})$$

Where $\rho_{uncured}$ is the density of the uncured composite and ρ_{cured} (ρ_d) is the density of the cured composite.

3.1.2.2. Water Sorption and Solubility

In the aqueous oral environment the dental composites absorb water and release unreacted monomers. Water sorption occurs mainly as a direct absorption by the polymer matrix. The glass filler will not absorb water into the bulk of the composite but can absorb water onto its surface. Thus, the amount of water sorption is depended on the matrix of the composite and the quality of the bond between the matrix and the filler. As such the value for the water sorption must be related to the matrix structure and content of the composite.

Water or solvent uptake into the matrix phase of composites causes two opposing processes. The solvent will extract unreacted components mainly monomers resulting in shrinkage, loss in weight and reduction of mechanical properties. Conversely solvent uptake leads to a swelling of the composite and an increase of weight. The solvent diffuses into the polymer network and separates the chains, creating an expansion. However since the polymer network contains microvoids created during polymerization and free volume between chains, a part of the solvent is accommodated without creating a change in volume. Thus the dimensional change of a polymer composite in a solvent is complex and difficult to predict and depends on the chemical structure of the matrix. The hydrophilicity of the matrix needs to be of sufficient magnitude to distend the matrix. In addition the mean elastic modulus of the polymer needs to be sufficient low to accommodate the distension. Hence the ratio between the elastic modulus of the polymer and the strength of its hydrophilic attraction may determine the capacity to alter the dimensions of the polymer. Expansion resulting from water sorption can be a clinically desirable phenomenon if it fully counteracts the effects of shrinkage. A coefficient of expansion that exceeds the shrinkage value is not desirable, as further stresses may be introduced into the teeth [60].

Usually the polymer matrix in current dental composites is prepared by copolymerization of two or more dimethacrylates such as Bis-GMA, Bis-EMA or UDMA (characterized as base monomers) with D_3MA or TEGDMA (characterized as diluents) (Figure 3. 2). The sorption of water by these glassy polydimethacrylates is generally described by a dual-mode theory, which assumes that the amount of the sorbed molecules consists of two populations. One is held by ordinary dissolution in the polymer matrix according to the Henry's law and the second is trapped in polymer microvoids following the Langmuir isotherm. A clear physical picture of this behaviour is described by the free volume theory, which suggests that glassy polymers generally have a non-equilibrium liquid structure containing an equilibrium hole-free volume responsible for Henry's sorption and an extra non-equilibrium hole-free volume, frozen into the polymer (micro-voids) responsible for Langmuir's sorption. The total hole-free volume effective for water diffusion depends on the macromolecular packing density. Flexible polymer chains with polar groups, especially those forming hydrogen bonds, which increase the intermolecular attractions favour high packing density. The sorbed water which is molecularly dispersed into the polymer matrix acts as plasticizer, causing the swelling of polymer. The quantity of thus sorbed water depends on the available equilibrium hole-free volume, the physicochemical affinity of polymer groups to water and the resistance of polymer chains to a swelling deformation stress. On the contrary the water molecules which are accommodated in micro-voids are hydrogen-bonded form clusters and do not cause swelling of polymer but act rather as filler particles.

The study of the water sorption of neat polymers made by light-curing of Bis-GMA, TEGDMA, UDMA or Bis-EMA showed that poly-TEGDMA absorbs the highest amount of water (6.33 wt%) and releases the lowest amount of unreacted monomer (2.41 μg/mm^3). Poly- Bis-EMA absorbs the lowest water amount (1.79 wt%) and releases the highest amount of unreacted monomer (14.21 μg/mm^3). Poly-UDMA absorbs 2.59 wt% and releases 6.62 μg/mm^3 of unreacted monomer. Poly-Bis-GMA absorbs 2.93 wt% and releases 10.44 μg/mm^3 of unreacted monomer. [60].

It is worth to note that according to ISO 9000s standard for dental restorative resins a resin in order to be suitable for use as dental material must show water sorption lower than 50 μg/mm^3 and solubility lower than 5 μg/mm^3. The values of water sorption for all studied polymers, expect that prepared from TEGDMA are within the range of the ISO's standard. On the contrary the values of solubility are within the range of the ISO's standard only for copolymers prepared from mixtures of Bis-GMA and TEGDMA. Z100 and Filtek Z250 are two current commercial composites the matrix resin of which consists correspondingly of copolymer Bis-GMA/TEGDMA and Bis-GMA/Bis-EMA/UDMA. The water sorption and solubility of these composites was found to be 16.85 μg/mm^3 (water sorption) and 0.73 μg/mm^3 (solubility) for Z100 and 13.02 μg/mm^3 (water sorption) and 0.25 μg/mm^3 (solubility) for Filtek Z250 [60].

The water uptake characteristics and solubility of polymers and commercial composites (Sculpt-It and Alert) based on Bis-EMA and a polycarbonate dimethacrylate (PCDMA) were also studied in detail in our lab [61]. The equilibrium water uptake from all copolymers Bis-EMA/PCDMA was very small with a trend to increase as the amount of PCDMA was increased. The inverse effect was observed in the solubility values. The composites studied exhibited also very low water uptake values in comparison to other composites reported in literature. Concerning the sorption rate data, it was observed that the polymers followed Fickian diffusion during almost whole sorption or desorption curve, while the composites showed this behaviour until only $M_t/M_\infty \approx 0.5$. The diffusion coefficients calculated for the polymers were larger than those of the composites and always higher during desorption compared to sorption. The values of the diffusion coefficients for both resins and composites were in the same order of magnitude with the values of the corresponding materials reported in the literature.

In a next work we have studied the sorption kinetics of 75 vol% ethanol/water solution, a well known food simulating liquid, by dimethacrylate- based dental resins and resin composites [62]. We found that the rate of the solution sorption follows Fickian diffusion kinetics during almost the whole sorption curve. According to Fick's Law the equation for diffusion in one dimension (χ) when the diffusion coefficient D is constant is expressed as:

$$\frac{\partial C}{\partial t} = D\frac{\partial^2 C}{\partial x^2}$$

in which C is the concentration of the diffusing species at time t

For a plane sheet geometry and if the initial concentration of the diffusing material is uniform and the surface is kept at concentration Co the above equation has a solution in the following form:

$$\frac{M_t}{M_\infty} = 1 - \frac{8}{\pi^2}\sum_{n=0}^{\infty}\frac{1}{(2n+1)^2}\exp\left(-\frac{(2n+1)^2\pi^2}{L^2}Dt\right)$$

Where L is the thickness of the specimen and M_t and M_∞ are the masses of solution sorbed at times t and ∞ respectively.

Accordingly for small times when M_t/M_∞ is small enough (<0.50), this equation is reduced to the equation:

$$\frac{M_t}{M_\infty} = \frac{4}{L}\left(\frac{Dt}{\pi}\right)^{1/2}$$

Table 3.6. Diffusion coefficients of net resins and the composites during sorption of 75vol% ethanol/water solution 37°C [62]

Material	Diffusion coefficients (10^8 cm^2 s^{-1})
Bis-GMA	2.4
TEGDMA	0.5
UDMA	1.5
Bis-EMA	2.9
Bis-GMA/TEGDMA (50/50 wt/wt)	0.4
Bis-GMA/TEGDMA (70/30 wt/wt)	0.4
Bis-GMA/UDMA/Bis-EMA	1.3
Z-100 MP	0.28
Filtek Z-250	0.18

From which, if one plots M_t/M_∞ against $t^{1/2}/L$ the diffusion coefficient can be calculated from the initial curve slope, using the so-called Stephan's approximation.

For all polymers and composites studied in our work [62] the initial part of the rate of ethanol/water sorption curves (i.e. until $M_t/M_\infty<0.5$) is always linear. Thus from the slope of these lines and applying the above equation the diffusion coefficient was calculated. Values of *D* for all specimens studied are shown in Table 3.6.

For the Fickian sorption of binary liquid mixtures as for example the 75vol% ethanol/water solution in methacrylate-based biomaterials in the form of thin sheets, a new iterative method was developed permitting the simultaneous determination of the self-diffusion coefficients of the components of the mixture and their uptake fractions at the equilibrium [63]. The approach is based on a new equation describing a parallel Fickian sorption of the components into thin polymer sheets. The procedure was tested with ideal and Monte Carlo simulated data. The method, applied to ideal simulated data that corresponded to various values of D_1, D_2 and *f* perfectly extracted the desired parameters. The application of the method to Monte Carlo simulated data revealed that this method is fairly applicable even when the simulated data are considerable obscured by "noise". Finally the proposed iterative method was successfully applied to the experimental data concerning the sorption kinetics of ethanol-water mixture (75vol% in ethanol) in thin poly-TEGDMA discs. The obtained values are equal to $D_{water} = 2.75\text{x}10^{-11}$ m^2s^{-1}, D_{EtOH}=$10.72\text{x}10^{-13}$ $m^2s^{-1}$and *f* %(percentage of the absorbed water) = 7.52 [63].

Despite the fact that the proposed iterative method requires laborious calculations, it can be easily applied thanks to the opportunities offered today by high speed personal computers. Thus using a common computer the extraction of the desired parameters (D_1, D_2, *f*) from a sorption curve requires only a few minutes. Finally it should be noted that the present procedure was designated to be applied to the sorption of ethanol-water mixture in methacrylate based biomaterials. However there is no reason why the proposed analysis could not be applied to the Fickian sorption of any binary mixtures in any polymer matrix [63].

On continuation of our work on this topic we have proposed two new methods the iterative and the graphical for the determination of self –diffusion coefficient (*D*) of water in methacrylate based biomaterials followed Fickian sorption [64]. The *D* value is traditionally determined by means of the initial slope of the corresponding sorption curve and the so-called Stefan's approximation. The proposed methods using equations without approximations and data resulting from the whole sorption range reach to accurate values of D even when the sorption curve does not present an initial linear portion. In addition to D the Graphical method allows the extrapolation of the mass of the sorbed water at equilibrium (M_∞) even when the equilibrium specimen's mass fluctuates around its limited value (m_∞). The test of the proposed procedures by means of ideal and Monte Carlo simulated data revealed that these methods are fairly applicable. The obtained D values compared with those determined by means of the Stephan's method revealed that the proposed methods provide more accurate results.

Based on this iterative method the sorbed and desorbed water or ethanol at equilibrium, the corresponding diffusion coefficients and the solubility were determined in dental resins prepared by light-curing of Bis-GMA, Bis-EMA, UDMA, TEGDMA or D_3MA [65]. Two cycles of sorption/desorption of water or ethanol by each resin were performed. The experimental curves $m_t=f(t)$ taken for the first water sorption by poly-Bis-GMA, poly-Bis-EMA, and poly-UDMA showed a maximum a maximum was also observed in the curve obtained for first sorption of ethanolby poly-Bis-GMA. In all other cases the curves foe sorption or desorption of water or ethanol showed Fickian behaviour. This maximum was attributed to the synergistic effect of the water sorption and the simultaneous desorption of the unreacted monomer. A new equation describing this effect was produced. The fitting of this equation to the experimental data allowed us to determine the diffusion coefficient of the water, the water % uptake at equilibrium, as well as the extracted mass of the unreacted monomer (solubility). Also in all cases it was shown that the determined parameters WS_1 and D_{S1} are apparent percentage magnitudes. The first quantity expresses the apparent percentage of the absorbed water or ethanol while the second quantity is related to the water diffusion coefficient during its sorption process, as well as to the diffusion coefficient of the monomer extraction. The actual value of water sorbed is expressed by parameter $WD_1=WD_2$ (water desorbed during first and second desorption). Based on this parameter the studied resins follow the order: TEGDMA>Bis-GMA>UDMA>Bis-EMA>D_3MA. Unreacted monomer is mainly extracted by water during the first sorption ($SL_1\%>>SL_2\%$). Comparison of the values of SL_1 % obtained for various resins in water show the following order: Bis-GMA>Bis-EMA≈UDMA>>TEGDMA> D_3MA.

Ethanol extracts also unreacted monomer during the first sorption ans so the determined values ES_1 and D_{S1} are apparent values. The amount of ethanol sorbed by resins is expressed by the parameters: $ES_2=ED_2=ED_1$. Based on this parameter the resins follow the order: Bis-GMA>UDMA>TEGDMA>D_3MA>Bis-EMA. This order is completely different from the order found in the case of water, indicating that the sorbed water or ethanol depends both on the resin and the solvent structure. The solubility of renins in ethanol follows the order: Bis-GMA>>UDMA> D_3MA>Bis-EMA>TEGDMA.

Also it was found that for poly-Bis-GMA and poly-D_3MA the solubility SL_1% in ethanol is much higher than the sum of solubility (SL_1+SL_2%) in water, which indicates that water does not extract all the amount of unreacted monomer even during the second sorption. In poly-Bis-EMA and poly-UDMA SL_1 in ethanol is almost equal to SL_1 in water.

As far as the diffusion the diffusion coefficient is concerned it was found to be indenpedent of the amount of water or ethanol sorbed. Poly-D_3MA showed low water or ethanol uptake but the highest diffusion coefficient for both water and ethanol sorption indicating that this process is governed by the formation of hydrogen bonds at polar sites [65].

In a next work we have determined the volumetric change of resins prepared by light curing of Bis-GMA, Bis-EMA, UDMA,TEGDMA or D_3MA after immersion in water or ethanol 37°C for 30 days [66]. Sorption and solubility tests were determined according to the method described in ANSI/ADA Specification No. 27-1993 or ISO 4049-1998. Specimen discs were prepared by filling a Teflon mould (15 mm in diameter and 1 mm in thickness) with the unpolymerized material, taking care to minimize entrapped air. The upper and lower surface of the mould was overlaid with glass slides. The completed assembly was held together with spring clips and irradiated using a dental photocuring unit. This source consisted a 75 W tungsten halogen lamp, which emits radiation between 420-500 nm and has the maximum peak at 470 nm where absorbs also camphorquinone (λ_{max}=470 nm ε=3.8x10^4 cm^2/mol). Due to the large size of our specimen this unit was used without the light guide at a distance from the sample of approximately 0.8 cm. The curing intensity at the position of the sample measured with a curing light meter was 200 mV/ cm^2. The samples were irradiated for 200 s on each side; this is the total time of shorter intervals of 40 s. The irradiation time of 200 s was found to be the optimum for the curing of the resins under the experimental conditions used [7]. Four specimen discs were prepared for each resin. Then, the mould was dismantled and the resin was carefully removed by flexing the Teflon mould.

All polymerized resins were placed in a desiccator and transferred in a pre-conditioning oven at 37°C. After 24 h they were removed, stored in the desiccator for 1 h and weighted to an accuracy of ±0.0001 g using an analytical balance. This cycle was repeated until a constant mass (m_i) was obtained. Then each specimen was placed in the holder immersed in water and the displayed apparent weight was noted (m_w). This procedure was done with extreme care to ensure that no air bubbles adhered to the solid. The density of the dry specimen was calculated based on the Archimedes' principle as follows:

$$\rho_d = \rho_o [m_i /(m_i - m_w)] \tag{1}$$

In which ρ_o is the density of the water used as the immersion fluid.

Following, the discs were immersed in water or ethanol at 37°C for 30 days. Then each specimen was removed from the test tube, was dried by blotting with absorbent tissue, was placed on the balance and the displayed weight was noted (m_s). The same specimen was removed from the pan and placed in the holder immersed in water for the determination of the density of the saturated specimen ρ_s. The percentage weight increase of specimens, *WI* (%), was calculated using the following formulae:

$$WI\,(\%) = 100\,(m_s - m_i)/\,m_i \tag{2}$$

This is an apparent value for the liquid sorbed, because unreacted monomer is simultaneously extracted resulting to decrease of specimen weight.

For the determination of monomer extracted the samples were transferred to a drying oven maintained at 37°C. After a time period of 30 days, they weighted in air (m_d) and in water (m_w) for the determination of density of dry specimens (ρ_d). The amount of unreacted monomer which extracted by water or ethanol, during the immersion for 30 days, known as "solubility" of the resin in these solvents was calculated from the formulae:

$$SL(\%) = 100\,(m_i - m_d)/\,m_i \tag{3}$$

The percentage amount of water or ethanol absorbed is then given by the formulae:

$$WS\,(\%) \text{ or } ES\,(\%) = WI\,(\%) + SL(\%) \tag{4}$$

Furthermore, the % volume increase, *VI* (%), is calculated using the available data on densities of the dry (ρ_d) and saturated (ρ_s) specimens:

Table 3.4. Amount (wt/wt%) of Different Monomers eluted from dental polymers as a function of Irradiation time after 30 days in 75vol% ethanol/water solution 37°C [67]

Material	Irradiation Time	Bis-GMA	TEGDMA	UDMA	Bis-EMA
Bis-GMA	60	4.98±0.62			
	80	3.45±0.11[d]			
	100	3.36±0.06[d]			
TEGDMA	60		1.54±0.05[a]		
	80		0.62±0.37[b]		
	100		0.44±0.11[c]		
UDMA	60			2.81 ±0.08[a,d]	
	80			0.61±0.34 [b]	
	100			0.50±0.12 [c]	
Bis-EMA	60				10.1±1.3[d]
	80				1.13±0.75[a]
	100				0.58±0.35[c]
Bis-GMA/TEGDMA(50/50wt/wt)	60	0.31±0.03[e]	0.27±0.02		
	100	0.26±0.02[e]	0.20±0.03		
Bis-GMA/TEGDMA(70/30wt/wt)	60	0.97±0.29	0.21±0.02		
	100	0.63±0.08	0.11±0.02		
Bis-GMA/UDMA/Bis-EMA	60	0.97±0.22[d]		1.17±0.13 [d]	1.05±0.22[a]
	100	0.32±0.03		0.35±0.03	0.26±0.10

Mean values ± standard deviation of three replicates; tha values with the same letter a, b, c are not significantly different (p>0.05)

[d] Statistically different (p<0.05) from the value obtained at 6 days immersion period of the same monomer from the same material at the same irradiation time. Values with no superscript are not statistically different.

[e] Statistically not different from the value obtained at 60 days immersion

$$VI = [100\,(\rho_d - \rho_s) + w\,\rho_d] / \rho_s \qquad (5)$$

Where *w* represents the % water or ethanol sorbed (*WS* % or *ES* %). Using the above expression, the fraction of the liquid contributing to an increase in swelling (*f*) in dimensionless form, is expressed as:

$$f = (VI \,/\, w\, \rho_d)\rho_l \qquad (6)$$

In which ρ_l is used to denote the density of the absorbed liquid. Values of *f* range between the extreme cases in which the liquid contributes all its volume to the resin (*f*=1) to that in which it contributes nothing (*f*=0). The provisional significance given to (1-*f*) is that it corresponds to the fraction of absorbed liquid, which accommodated in microvoids without causing swelling.

In the case of water the polymers follow the order: poly-TEGDMA>poly-Bis-GMA>poly-UDMA>poly-Bis-EMA>poly-D_3MA. On the contrary the order in ethanol is poly-Bis-GMA > poly-UDMA> poly-TEGDMA >poly-Bis-EMA ≈ poly-D_3MA. The volume increase was found to depend linearly on the amount of water or ethanol absorbed [66].

Table 3.5. Amount (wt/wt%) of Different Monomers eluted from dental polymer composite as a function of irradiation time after 30 days in 75vol% ethanol/water solution 37°C [67]

	Irradiation				
Material	**Time**	**Bis-GMA**	**TEGDMA**	**UDMA**	**Bis-EMA**
Z-100 MP	40	0.044±0.010 (0.23)	0.093±0.013(0.49)		
	60	0.038±0.006 (0.20)	0.073±0.012(0.38)		
Filtek Z-250	20	0.153±0.010 (0.66)	0.066±0.004(0.28)	2.480±0.078[a] (10.8)	0.236±0.020[a](1.02)
	60	0.098±0.011 (0.43)	0.061±0.005(0.26)	1.484±0.094[a] (6.5)	0.135±0.08[a] (0.59)

The values in parentheses express the wt/wt-% on the organic matrix content. Mean values± standard deviation of three replicates.

[a] Statistically different (p<0.05) from the value obtained at 6 days immersion period of the same monomer from the same material at the same irradiation time. Values with no superscript are not statistically different.

Solubility measurements in dental biomaterials reflect the leachable by the water amount of the unreacted monomer. This is trapped during the polymerization inside the microgels between the polymer chains and is absorbed to the surrounding network or it is trapped in micropores (monomer pools). The monomer in micropores is more susceptible to leaching out than the monomer inside the microgels [60].

In our lab we have studied the elution of residual monomers from light-cured dental resins and resin composites into a 75 vol% ethanol /water solution using High-Performance Liquid Chromatography (HPLC) [67]. The resins studied were made by light curing of Bis-GMA, TEGDMA, UDMA or Bis-EMA and mixtures of these monomers. The resin composites were made from two commercial light cured restorative materials (Z100 MP and Filtek Z250) the resin matrix of which is based on copolymers of these monomers. The 75 vol% ethanol /water solution was used because US FDA recommends the use of this solution as a food/oral simulating liquid. In this study resins and resin composites were fabricated under the same experimental conditions (specimen size, light curing intensity and time) and immersed in the 75 vol% ethanol /water solution at 37°C for certain time intervals. The amount of different monomers eluted (wt/wt-%) from the resins as a function of irradiation time after 30 days immersion in the ethanol solution determined by HPLC is presented in Table 3.4. Correspondingly, the amount of different monomers eluted (wt/wt-%) from the polymer composites as a function of irradiation time after 30 days immersion in the solution is presented in Table 3.5. For all the materials studied it was observed that thethe chemical structure of the monomers used for the preparation of resins, which defines the chemical and physical structure of the corresponding resin directly affects the amount of eluted monomers, as well as the time needed for the elution of this amount. In the case of composites it seems that the elution process it is not influenced by the presence of filler.

3.1.2.3. Thermal Properties

Thermal expansion is a crucial factor that challenges the adhesive bond between restorations and tooth structure. A great difference in the coefficient of linear thermal expansion (CLTE) between tooth and the restorative material leads to different dimensional changes occurring when there is a temperature change in the restored tooth. Such expansions and contractions develop stresses at the tooth-restorative interface, which may lead to the formation of microleakages at the margins of the restoration. The penetration of acid and microorganisms can result in the Pulpal damage can result from toxic products liberated by microorganisms. Staining can occur at the margin of the restoration resulting from accumulation of debris. Also there is a strong correlation between microleakages and the coefficient of linear thermal expansion. Of course the failure of an adhesive bond is complex and is depended by a number of factors; however the driving force was found to be the difference in the CLTE between tooth structure and restoration. It is for this reason that ideally restorative materials should have similar coefficients of thermal expansion to enamel and dentine of tooth. For various commercial polymer composites this coefficient was found to range from 26 to $35x10^{-6}/^oC$ or from 26 to $83.5x10^{-6}/^oC$ or from 20 to $80x10^{-6}/^oC$; all for the temperature range 0-60°C. For the enamel and dentine it is $17x10^{-6}/^oC$ and about $11\ x10^{-6}/^oC$ respectively [17]. Since the thermal expansion of composites is greater than that of tooth structure composite restorations will have a greater change in dimensions with changes in oral temperatures than tooth structure will. The more the polymer matrix the higher is the linear coefficient of thermal expansion, since the polymer has a higher value than the filler [58].

The thermal expansion characteristics of dental resins prepared by light-curing of Bis-GMA, Bis-EMA, UDMA , TEGDMA and polycarbonate dimethacrylate (PCDMA) and of commercial light-cured resin composites (Z-100 MP, Filtek Z-250, Sculpt-It and Alert) the organic matrix resin of which is based on different combinations of the above monomers were studied recently in our lab by thermomechanical analysis (TMA) [68]. This study showed the existence of a glass-transition temperature (Tg) at around 35-47°C for the resins and 40-45 °C for the composites; then the coefficient of linear thermal expansion (CLTE) was calculated at the temperatures intervals 0-60 °C, 0-Tg and Tg-60 °C. The CLTE values of Bis-GMA, TEGDMA and UDMA resins are similar and lower than those of Bis-EMA and PCDMA resins. The CLTE values of the composites indicated that the major factor that affects the CLTE of a composite is the filler content, but it also seems to be affected by the chemical structure of the resin matrix. TMA on water-saturated samples showed that water desorption takes place during the measurement and that the residual water acts as a plasticizer decreasing the Tg and increasing the CLTE values.

The thermal conductivity of composite is much lower than that for metallic restorations and closely matches that of enamel and dentine. Therefore composites provide good thermal insulation for the dental pulp [58].

3.1.2.4. Radiopacity

Early composites were characteristically radiolucent because the filler was quartz and a clinical evaluation was conducted either by direct observation or by transillumination. Later composites included glasses having atoms with high atomic numbers such as barium, strontium and zirconium. The typical fillers such as quartz, lithium aluminum glasses and silica are not radiopaque and must be blended with other fillers to produce a radiopaque composite. Even at thir highest volume fraction of filler the amount of radiopacity seen in composites is noticeably less than exhibited by a metallic restorative like amalgam. Aluminum is used as a standard reference for radiopacity. A 2 mm thickness of dentin is equivalent in radiopacity to 2.5 mm of aluminum and enamel is equivalent to 4 mm of aluminum. To be effective a material should exceed the readiopacity of enamel but international standards accept radiopacity equivalent to 2 mm of aluminum. Amalgam has a radiopacity greater than 10 mm of aluminum which exceeds all the composite materials available [1].

3.1.2.5. Color

The color of an object is modified not only by the intensity and shade of the pigment or coloring agent but also by the translucency or opacity of the object. The body tissues vary in the degree of opacity that they exhibit. Most of them possess a degree of translucency. This is especially true of tooth enamel and the supporting soft tissues surrounding the teeth.

Opacity is a property of materials that prevents the passage of light. An opaque material may absorb some of the light and reflect the remainder. *Translucency* is a property of substances that permits the passage of light but disperses the light so that objects cannot be seen through the material. *Transparent* materials allow the passage of light in such a manner that little distortion takes place and objects may be clearly seen through them [1].

The earliest composites suffered from discoloration which can manifest itself in one of three ways:

- Marginal discoloration
- General surface discoloration
- Bulk discoloration

Marginal discoloration is usually due to the presence of a marginal gap between the restoration and the tooth tissues. Debris penetrates the gap and leads to an unsightly marginal stain; elimination of the marginal gap would completely avoid this type of staining. General surface discoloration may be related to the surface roughness of the composite and is more likely to occur with those composites employing large filler particles. Debris gets trapped in the spaces between the protruding filler particles and is not readily removed by tooth brushing. Polishing with a suitable abrasive should remove this surface stain [18].

3.1.2.6. Biocompatibility

Polymeric composites are complex structures and various components are released from them such as residual monomers, impurities of monomers, additives degradation products. These may irritate the soft tissue, stimulate the growth of bacteria and promote allergic reactions. The substances released from polymer composites and glass ionomer cements have been well reviewed recently by Geurtsen [69]. It was found that some of them showed in several *in vitro* studies cytotoxic, genotoxic, mutagenic or estrogenic effects and pulpal and gingival/oral mucosa reactions [70].

Acrylates and mainly methacrylates were found to cause cytotoxic effects. Evaluation of the cytotoxicity of 39 acrylates and methacrylates that have been in dental polymer composites showed a relationship between their structure and the degree of cytotoxicity. TEGDMA and mainly Bis-GMA and UDMA showed high cytoxicity. TEGDMA was found recently to be moderately mutagenic in V79 cells at subtoxic concentrations. Bis-GMA has also exhibited in low concentrations as 0.02 and 0.6 mM positive responses in DNA-synthesis inhibition test, which measures the mutagenic effects of substances in human genes. Furthermore it was reported that TEGDMA might promote the proliferation of the important cariogenic microorganisms *Lactobacillus acidophilus* and *Streptococcus sobrinus* [67].

3.1.2.7. Fluoride Release

The caries preventive effect of fluoride ions is proven and extensively documented. This can also be seen from the caries prevention methods resulting from this fact such as e.g. fluoridation of potable water and use of tooth pastes containing fluoride. Restorative materials containing fluoride ions, e.g. silicate cements and glass ionomer cements are also said to help prevent caries. On the basis of this knowledge efforts were made to achieve an anti-cariogenic potential also in composite restorative materials by adding fluorides. The requirements for such a composite may not only be limited to the highest possible content of releasable fluoride ions. It has to be proved and tested that the fluoride release has no negative effects, such as discolorations, or that the mechanical/physical properties of the restorative composite do not clearly deteriorate. Certainly the choice is restricted by these requirements to a few fluorides of low solubility [71].

3.1.2.8. Mechanical Properties

3.1.2.8.1. Compressive Strength

This is particularly important in the process of mastication because many of the forces of mastication are compressive. Compressive strength is most useful for comparing materials that are brittle and generally weak in tension and that as a result are not employed where tensile forces predominate. When a structure is subjected to compression, note that, the failure of the body may occur as a result of complex stress formations in the body. This illustrated by a cross-sectional view of a right cylinder subjected to compression as shown in Figure 3.20. It is apparent from this Figure that the forces of compression applied to each end of the sample are resolved into forces of shear along a cone-shaped area at each end and into tensile forces in the central portion of the mass as a result of the action of the two cones on the cylinder. Because of this resolution of forces in the body it has become necessary to adopt standard sizes and dimensions to obtain reproducible test results. Figure 3.20 shows that if a test sample is too short, the force distributions become more complicated as a result of the cone formations overlapping in the ends of the cylinder. If the sample is too long buckling may occur. Therefore for the most satisfactory results the cylinder should have a length approximately twice that of the diameter [1].

Compressive strenght (CS) in Megapascal is given by the equation:

$$CS=F/d^2$$

Where F is the maximum force in Newtons exerted on the specimen and d is the diameter of the specimen in millimeters.

3.1.2.8.2. Diametral Tensile Strength

An alternative method of testing brittle materials in which the ultimate tensile strength of a brittle material is determined through compressive testing has become popular, because of its relative simplicity and reproducibility of results. The method is described in the literature as the diametral compression test for tension, the Brazilian test or the indirect tensile test. In this test method a disk of the brittle material is compressed diametrically in a testing machine until fracture occurs.

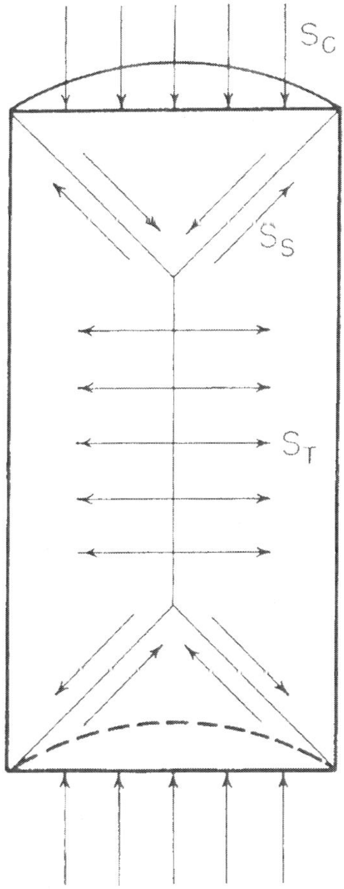

Figure 3.20. Drawing of complex stress pattern developed in cylinder subjected to compressive stress [1].

3.1.2.8.3. Flexural Strength and Modulus of Elasticity

Particularly with restorations which demonstrate thin layers and/or are supported only by little or no tooth substance, high twisting forces arise. The flexural strength of a material indicates how much force is necessary to break a test specimen. The distortion under load in form of modulus of elasticity is simultaneously measured during these measurements. A lower modulus of elasticity means high distortion which is an undesirable property in dental composites. If high flexural strength is only reached through creating a material that gives way too easily which compromises the strength, then an unnatural load distribution results from chewing strength no longer being horizontally distributed over the paradentium. In this case, occlusal pressure constitutes a lateral tensile load on the surface which can lead to loss of adhesion on the cavity wall and thus marginal caries. In deeper regions within the cavity, the occlusal load on flexible filling materials induces a lateral expansion which can lead to breaks in the remaining lateral tooth surface. High flexural strength in combination with a tooth-like, high modulus of elasticity is desirable in every case.

In a recent work [72] we have determined the flexure and the tensile strength of the neat homopolymer resins prepared from Bis-GMA, UDMA or decanemethylene dimethacrylate (D_3MA); also of the neat copolymer resin prepared from Bis-GMA (65 wt%) UDMA (20 wt%) and D_3MA (15 wt%) and the commercial dental composite Heliomolar RO and the resin matrix of which consists of the copolymer BisGMA/UDMA/ D_3MA (65/20/15 w/w/w). Flexural strength and tensile strength tests were determined according to the method described in ADA Specification (No 27) or ISO 4049. For flexural strength test bar shaped specimens (2 mm x 2 mm x 25 mm) were prepared, while for the tensile strength test dump-bell-shaped specimens were prepared. Both tests were made with a mechanical testing machine (Instron Universal Testing Instrument Model 1122, Instron Co.). The flexural strength (σ) in MPa was calculated using the following equation:

$$\sigma=3Fl/2bh^2$$

where F represents the maximum load in N exerted on the specimen, l the distance in mm between the supports, h the height of specimen in mm measured immediately prior to testing and b is the width of specimen in mm measured prior to testing.

The tensile strength (TS) was calculated using the following equation

$$TS=F/dw$$

Where F represents the maximum force in N exerted on the specimen, d the depth of specimen in mm at the fracture surface and w is the width of specimen in mm at the fracture surface.

Samples of neat resins and Heliomolar RO prepared by light curing were also immersed in water or 75vol% ethanol/water 37 °C for 1, 7 or 30 days. Then the flexural and tensile strength were determined. Bis-GMA and copolymer resin did not showed any significant change in mechanical properties after immersion in water or 75vol% ethanol/water 37 °C for 30 days. On the contrary UDMA, D_3MA and the composite Heliomolar RO showed a significant decrease.

The modulus of elasticity is determined in a 3-point flexural strength test from the deflection of the material in relationship to the applied force. The modulus of elasticity is dominated by the amount of filler and increases exponentially with the volume fraction of filler. The elastic modulus represents the stiffness of a material within the elastic range. A low modulus indicates a flexible material. This stiffness is important in applications where high biting forces are involved and wear resistance is essential. The flexural modulus is measured by applying a load to a material specimen that is supported at each end.

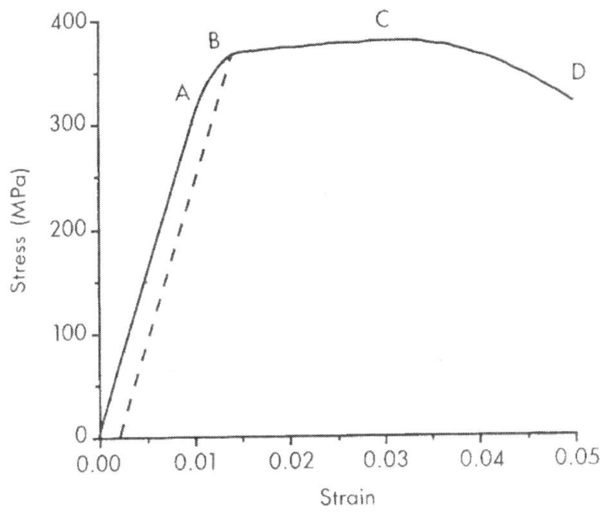

Figure 3.21. Stress-strain curve for a material subjected to a tensile stress.

3.1.2.8.4. Fracture Strength

The stress at which a material fractures is called the fracture strength or fracture stress. In Figure 3.21 the test sample fractured at point D at the end of the curve.

3.1.2.9. Dynamic Mechanical Properties

Although static properties frequently can be related to the function of a material under dynamic conditions, there are limitations to using the static properties to estimate the properties of materials subjected to dynamic loading. The mechanical properties of dental composites tranditionally have been investigated using static methods. However these focus only on the elastic component of the composite. Dental composites exhibit viscoelastic behaviour due to the presence of polymer matrix, which is a viscoelastic material. Dynamic tests such as dynamic mechanical analysis (DMA) on the other hand are particularly well suited for viscoelastic materials, since they determine both the elastic and viscous response of material. Also dynamic tests mimic better the cyclic masticatory loading to which dental composites are clinically subjected. This might be extremely valuable to predict the clinical performance of biomaterials when working performance of biomaterials when working under the cyclic solicitations generated by the human body's physiological movements.

DMA imposes a very small oscillating strain on a small amplitude stress-strain curves at a specified frequency. The force required to generate this strain in the specimen can be measured. The force which the specimen generates when it returns to its neutral position can also be determined. These forces can be converted into energy values by use of the known strain values. Purely elastic materials have stress and strain in phase, so that the response of one caused by the other is immediate. In purely viscous materials strain lags stress by a 90°C phase lag. Viscoelastic materials exhibit behavior somewhere in the middle of these two types of materials. The Young's storage modulus (E') is a measure of the energy stored elastically, whereas the Young's loss modulus (E'') is a measure of the energy lost as heat. The ratio of loss and storage modulus (E''/E'=tanδ) called tangent delta is a dimensionless parameter which conveys no physical magnitude, but is a measure of the ratio of energy lost to energy stored in a cyclic deformation. δ is the angle between the in phase and out of phase components in the cycle motion. Tan δ also goes through a maximum. The maximum in the E'' and tanδ are used for the determination of glass transition temperature (Tg).

The viscoelastic properties of several contemporary dental resin composites have been studied in our lab by using DMA. DMA is suggested as a valuable tool for characterization of viscoelasticity of dental composites giving a greater insight into their mechanical behavior. In our lab recently the viscoelastic properties (E', E'', tanδ, Tg) of current commercial dental resin composites have been studied by DMA [73,74].

3.1.2.10. Wear

Wear is the process by which material is displaced or removed by the interfacial forces which generated as two surfaces rub together. In the oral environment occur the following types of wear: (1) adhesive wear; (2) corrosive wear; (3) surface fatigue; (4) abrasive wear. *Adhesive wear* is characterized by the formation and disruption of microjunctions.

Corrosive wear is secondary to physical removal of a protective layer and is therefore related to the chemical activity of the wear surfaces. The sliding action of the surfaces removes any surface barriers and causes accelerated corrosion. In *fatigue wear* the repeated loading of teeth produces cyclic stresses that can in time lead to the growth of fatigue cracks. These cracks often form below the surface and initially grow parallel to it before veering towards the surface or coalescing with other cracks.

Abrasive wear involves a soft surface in contact with a harder surface. In this type of wear particles are pulled off of one surface and adhere to the other during sliding. When two surfaces rub together, the harder of the two materials may indent, produce grooves in, or cut away material from the other surface. This direct contact wear is known as *two-body abrasion* and occurs in the mouth whenever there is direct tooth-to-tooth contact in what most dentists would call *attrition*. Abrasive wear may also occur when there is an abrasive slurry interposed between two surfaces such that the two solid surfaces are not actually in contact. This is called *three-body abrasion* and occurs in the mouth during mastication with food acting as the abrasive agent.

3.1.2.11. Hardness

The surface hardness of a dental material can be measured readily by a number of techniques resulting in a hardness value that can be used to compare different composites. Some of the most common methods of testing the hardness of restorative materials are the Brinell, Knoop, Vickers, Rockwell and Shore A hardness tests. Each of these tests differs slightly from the others and each prevents certain advantages and disadvantages. The various hardness tests differ in the indenter material, geometry and load. The choice of a hardness test depends on the material of interest the expected hardness range and the desired degree of localization.

The general procedure for testing hardness independent of the specific test is as follows. A standardized force or weight is applied to the penetrating point. Such a force application to the indenter produces a symmetrically shaped indentation which can be measured under a microscope for depth, area or width of indentation produced. The indentation dimensions are then related to tabulated hardness values. With a fixed load applied to a standardized indenter the dimensions of the indentation vary inversely with the resistance to penetration of the material tested. Thus lighter loads are needed for softer materials [1]

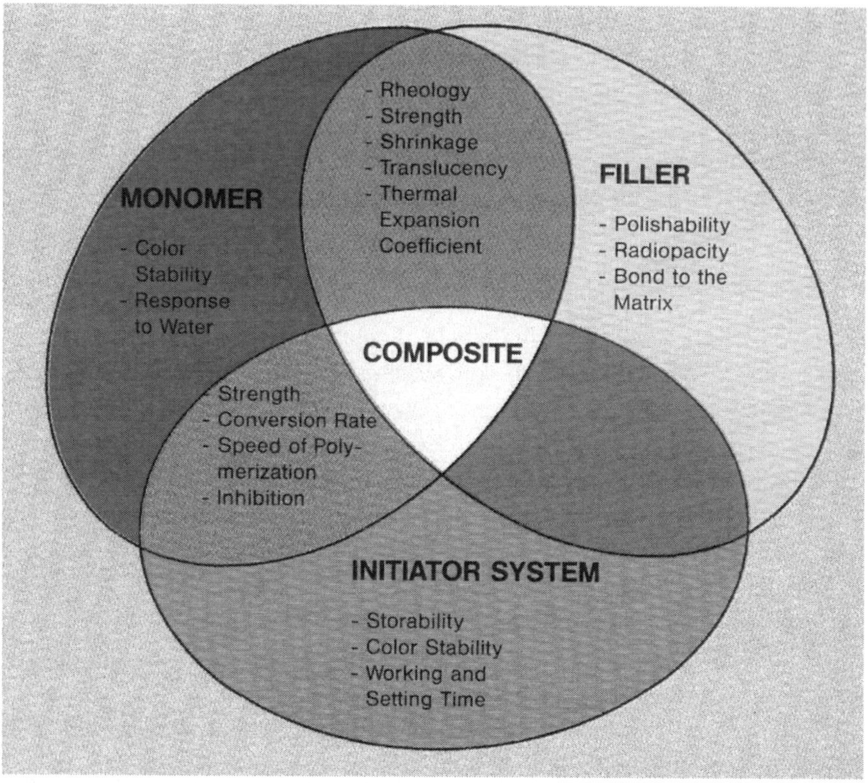

Figure 3.22. Interaction of the components of a dental polymer composite.

3.1.3. Interaction of Components-General Aspects

The individual components of dental polymer composites influence one another. The sum of these interdependent reactions produces the composite with its specific characteristics. Therefore no single property of the polymer composite can be changed without influencing the other features. A simplified graphic representation of some of these interactions between components is shown in Figure 3.22.

3.1.3.1. Interaction Monomer-Filler

Properties such as compressive strength, bending strength and hardness are controlled by the filler level, the filler type, their combinations and the monomers used. Higher filler levels increase the values for physical properties such as compressive strength or hardness and generally reduce water absorption. The size and form of the filler particles influence these values as well. Monomers or mixtures of monomers also have an effect on physical strength as well as characteristics of water absorption, conversion rate and the speed of polymerization. The relationships are sometimes vague and not all properties can be optimized with a single monomer mixture. Compromises must usually be found to reach the best possible balance of characteristics.

The rheology or consistency of a composite is determined by the viscosity of the monomers together with the filler level and the particle size. Fine filler particles produce tough and sticky composites while larger fillers make the composites drier and more dough-like. Acceptable consistencies are achieved by combinations of filler sizes.

The reason for the polymerization shrinkage is the larger distance between the double-bonded carbons (C=C) of adjacent monomers than the distance between polymerized monomer molecules. Monomers react to form polymer chains reducing the intermolecular distance and increasing the density. Shrinkage correlates directly with the number of reacted double bonds. Polymerization shrinkage can be reduced by reducing the proportion of monomer or by utilizing monomers with a high molecular weight. These monomers have a high viscosity and cannot be filled to the same high levels as monomers with low viscosity. A high filler level has often been "purchased" with a low molecular weight monomer the cost is a composite with a higher shrinkage.

The transparency of a composite is determined by the particle size of the filler and by the correlation of the refractive indices of the individual components. A high transparency is produced when the filler and polymer have the same refractive index. Very fine particles (under 0.2 microns) and very large particles (over 10 microns) aid in achieving a high transparency. Particle sizes between 0.2 and 10 microns are unfavorable.

Most fillers have a coefficient of thermal expansion similar to natural tooth substance. Polymers on the other hand have much higher expansion coefficients. The filler level is decisive for the thermal coefficient of the polymer composite [71,75].

3.2. Pit and Fissure Sealants

Which is the proper term: tooth sealants, dental sealants, or pit and fissure sealants? It really doesn't matter which of the phrases, tooth sealants, dental sealants, or pit and fissure sealants, you use when discussing matters with your dentist. To them, all of these terms are synonymous. If you mention any one of them, they will know precisely what you mean. The technique of utilizing tooth sealants as a way to protect teeth from tooth decay has been around for a long time, in fact for over a generation. The groundwork research for tooth sealants was laid back in the 1950's and 1960's. The first commercially available tooth sealants were marketed to dentists in the early 1970's [76].

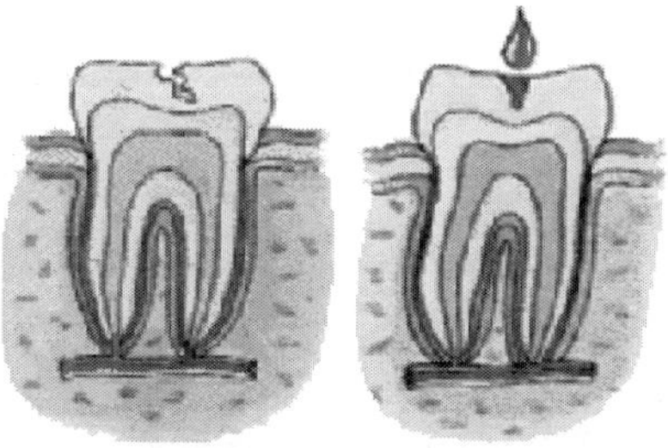

Pit and fissure sealants, are made of a thin plastic material that is applied to the chewing surfaces of the back teeth — premolars and molars. The chewing surfaces of molars and premolars are not smooth. They have pits and fissures where the toothbrush bristles can't reach. So, dental plaque is free to grow causing tooth decay (even with good dental hygiene). Most of the cavities on a kid's freshly erupted permanent teeth occur in these areas. Dental caries research have revealed that almost 84% of caries in ages 5-17 involved these pit and fissure areas [77]. There are four different types of teeth in the mouth of an adult human. The complete dentition of an adult person has 32 teeth (Figure 3.23) [78]. The adult human teeth show a morphology mainly differentiated by the shape of their upper surface (crown) and the number of the tooth roots. Individual tooth morphology is associated with the purpose of each tooth type (cutting, shredding or grinding the food). The four different types of human teeth are:

1) INCISORS or Cutting teeth

2) The 8 incisors are the very front human teeth with rather flat surfaces, a straight sharp horizontal edge for cutting and biting the food and one long, single, conical root.
3) CANINE teeth

   The 4 canine teeth are very strong, pointed corner teeth for tearing and shredding, placed laterally to each lateral incisor. They are larger and stronger than the incisors. The canine tooth morphology is characterized by the large, conical crown which projects beyond the level of the other teeth and one single root, longer than all other human teeth types. The upper canine teeth are sometimes called eyeteeth.
4) PREMOLARS or Bicuspid teeth.

   The 8 premolars, used for the chewing of the food, are placed lateral to and behind the canine teeth, with a flat upper surface and 1-2 roots. Their crown has two pyramidal eminences or cusps.
5) MOLARS or Molar teeth

   The 12 molars are the back human teeth. Molar teeth have a much different tooth morphology with large and flat upper surface and 2-4 roots. Molars is the one of types of teeth with the largest of the permanent teeth, used for the final chewing and grinding of the food before swallowing. (mola is the latin word for mill).The third molars are also known as wisdom teeth.

Buonocore's classic study of 1955 marked the start of a major revolution in the clinical practice of dentistry [79]. The first clinical benefit from Buonocore's work was the introduction of the first dental pit and fissure sealant, Nuva-Seal (L.D. Caulk) in February 1971, along with its curing initiator and ultraviolet light source, the Caulk Nuva Lite. However it took several more years before the sealant technique began to be adopted in clinical dentistry to any significant degree. Even now, almost 30 years after the introduction of pit and fissure sealants to the dental market place, the profession has not embraced the procedure to the extent that available scientific data would lead one to expect [80].

The sealant is a mixture of vinyl monomers, which can be polymerized by a free radical polymerization and has a viscosity low enough to penetrate into narrow pits and fissures easily and can be cured in them to become a hard and durable sealing material. Bis-GMA, its homologues and urethane dimethacrylate (UDMA) are very popular as the main monomer for polymer sealants and they are usually used together with other monomers that are less viscous, such as TEGDMA, in order to increase their penetration ability. Pits and fissures are treated with phosphoric acid, citric acid or other acidic agents prior to application of sealants. This treatment often called "acid etching" changes the enamel surface to a micro-rugged structure, which aids penetration of sealants into fissures and results in micromechanical adhesion between sealants and tooth substances. Acidic monomers have been introduced into the chemical formulation of sealants to further enhance the adhesion and penetration into fissures [81].

Polymerization of sealants is initiated by a redox system or by light irradiation. In the former case, benzoylperoxide/amine is most common and sulfinates also are used when acidic monomers are contained. [82]. Commercial products are composed of two liquid components: one has benzoyl peroxide and the other has an amine. In the latter case visible light is irradiated to initiate radical polymerization. Camphorquinone is the most popular photosensitizer and is usually used together with some kinds of amines [83]. Light cured sealants have one liquid component.

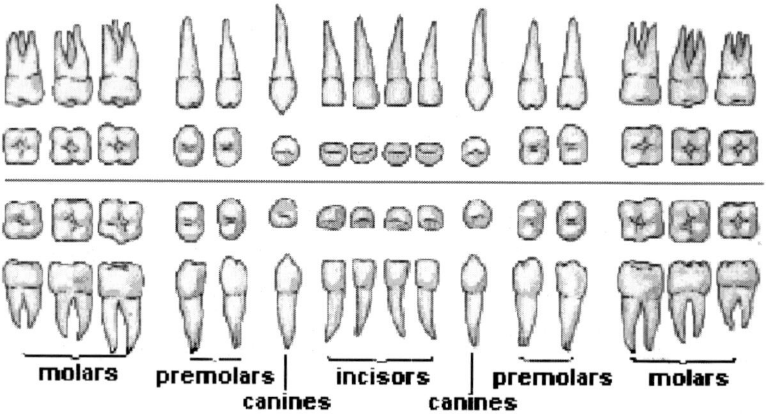

Figure 3.23. The picture of adult human teeth.

Manipulation of pit and fissures polymer sealants is simple. Once one drop of a sealant is placed onto any part of acid-etched pit and fissure, sealant quickly runs along fissure and penetrates into it by capillary action. Photopolymerizable sealants can be cured by the 10-30s of visible light irradiation, and redox curing sealants harden within 3-5 min after the two liquid components are mixed. There are some sealants that can release fluoride ion gradually. Fluoride ion converts hydroxyapatite, the major inorganic component of teeth to fluoroapatite, which is more acid-resistant than hydroxyapatite, reducing caries susceptibility.

Fluoride release technology, which is increasingly used, requires application of microencapsulated sodium fluoride and application of copolymer of methyl methacrylate and methacrylic fluoride. [84]. In the latter case, acid fluoride is embedded in the cured sealant; it reacts with water, which slowly permeates into the polymer network of the sealant and releases fluoride ion gradually.

3.3. ADHESIVES

Adhesion occurs when two unlike substances join together on being brought into contact, because of forces of attraction between them. Distinguish this from *cohesion* which results from attraction between like molecules. An *adhesive* is a material used to produce adhesion. The *adherend* is the substance to which the adhesive is applied.

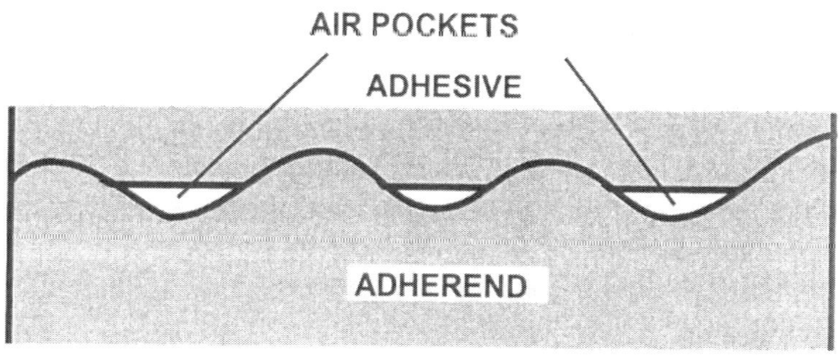

Figure 3.24. Air trapped between adhesive and adherend.

Two mechanisms of bonding are possible, either or both of which may operate [85]:

1) Chemical adhesion occurs if chemisorption occurs.
2) Micromechanical adhesion or attachment occurs when a liquid flows into pores or crevices in the adherend surface. When the fluid sets, micromechanical interlocking occurs producing a potentially strong bond

To obtain good adhesion, a number of factors are important. Good wetting of the adherend by the adhesive is important. Surface texture must be suitable; micromechanical adhesion requires a roughened surface on the adherend. The adherent surface must be clean and free of debris. Contaminated surfaces usually have critical surface tension values, so will not be capable of being wetted as easily as clean surfaces. The adhesive must have a suitable viscosity to enable it to flow readily over the surface of the adherend. Air pockets between adhesive and adherend be avoided (Figure 3.24) [85].

The primary aim of dental adhesives is to provide a strong bond between the filling material and the natural tooth substance (enamel and dentin). Dentin forms the bulk of the tooth and is found inside the enamel exterior. By volume dentin is of 50% carbonated apatite, 30% organic collagen and 20% fluid. Dentin has a tubular structure which becomes important in surface preparation and bonding. Most adhesive systems depend on the modification of the dentine surface for adhesive penetration and achievement of a strong bond. Bonding occurs partially through chemical bonding and partially through mechanical interlocking [86]. Researchers have used a great number of reactive chemical compounds as dental adhesive monomers. However, many of the commercially available enamel-dentin adhesives are very technique sensitive and show limited storage stability at ambient temperature. In recent years a new generation of easy- to- handle one bottle self-etching enamel-dentin adhesives was developed.

Self-etching enamel-dentin adhesives are based on the use of polymerizable, strongly acidity monomers that simultaneously condition and prime the enamel and dentin. The clinical requirements for self-etching enamel-dentin adhesives involve the removal of the weak smear layer on top of the dentin and creation of an adequate etch pattern on the enamel in a clinically relevant period of time (i.e., 15-30 s). Inward diffusion of comonomers into etched enamel and dentin followed by the polymerization under formation of resin-tags and of the so-called hybrid layer are responsible for strong bonds between the cured adhesive layer and the dental hard tissues [87].

The monomers used in commercial self-etching adhesives can be dived into three main categories according to their function: a) self-etching adhesive monomers b) cross-linking monomers and c) additional monofunctional comonomers (Figure 3.25).

All these monomers have to meet the following general requirements [87,88]:

- A high rate of free-radical homo- or copolymerization with the other monomers in the adhesive.
- The monomers should be advantageously miscible both with aqueous solutions of acetone or ethanol, which are mainly used as solvents in commercial self-etching adhesives and the other used monomers and additives.

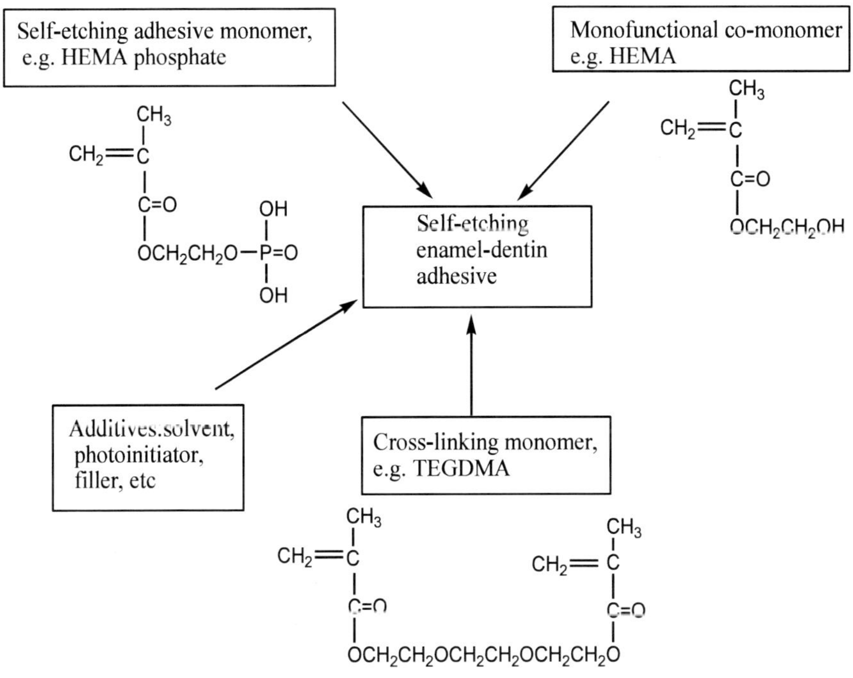

Figure 3.25. Components of currently available self-etching enamel dentin adhesives [87,88].

- Sufficient stability of both the monomer and the formed polymer. The monomer stability includes not only stability against premature polymerization, but also the hydrolytic stability in water during storage.
- Minimal water uptake and low swelling degree of the formed polymer and the monomers should not impair sufficient mechanical strength of the adhesive layer.

- Low oral toxicity and cytotoxicity of the monomers; they must show any mutagenic or carcinogenic effect with or without metabolic activation.

These general requirements can be fulfilled with structure-designed monomers containing one or more polymerizable groups and additional functional groups which are combined by a tailor made spacer group. Different kinds of polymerizable groups and hence resin systems exist (Figure 3.27). Acrylates and especially methacrylates monomers are most common. In general the advantages of acrylic systems are an easy radical polymerization reaction and their colourless and tasteless character [89]. The main difference between acrylates and methacrylates (one additional methyl- group) is their reactivity. In contrast to methacrylates the double bond of acrylates are much more reactive and may therefore pose biocompatibility and self-life problems [90]. Moreover methacrylates are also less sensitive to oxygen inhibition [91]. Both acrylates and methacrylates are vulnerable to water degradation (hydrolysis) of the ester group (R_1-CO-OR_2) [92]. A new group of monomers, methacrylamides have an amide group (R_1-CO-NH-R_2) instead of an ester group, which is more resistant to water [88,93,94]. Vinyl or styryl derivatives are less reactive (Figure 3.26). Moreover in the case of allyl or 1,2-disubstituted ethylene derivatives, such as maleic acid polymerization takes place only in the presence of more reactive cross-linking monomers [95]. Considering polarity, the polymerizable group generally exhibits hydrophobic behaviour.

The spacer of the adhesive monomer does not have a function as such, except for keeping both functional and polymerizable groups well separated, but it has an important influence on the properties of the monomer and the resulting polymer [96].The spacer is usually an alkyl-chain but can also contain several other groups, like esters, amides or aromatic groups. The polarity of the spacer will partly determine the solubility of the monomer in water and other solvents. The hydroplilicity of the spacer group may also cause water uptake, which leads to higher hydrolysis susceptibility of the monomers as well as swelling and discoloration of the cured resin. The size of the spacer group determines the viscosity of the monomer and as a consequence also its wetting and penetration behaviour. In addition small monomers will be more volatile than larger molecules [90]. The spacer also influences the flexibility of the monomer. Moreover, stereochemic and substituent effects by the spacer will modify the reactivity of polymerizable and/or functional groups [89]. Voluminous groups may cause other monomers not to reach the polymerizable group, there by hindering good polymerization (steric hindering) [89]. It has been shown in homopolymerization studies that the reactivity of monomers increases with increasing distance between the methacrylate groups [90] and the flexibility of the spacer of the monomer [97].

Self-etching adhesive monomers are monomer components in a self-etching enamel-dentin adhesive, which are responsible for the specific interaction of the adhesive with the dental hard tissue. Therefore they should meet, beside the above mentioned general requirements, the following additional demands [88]:

- Capability of self-etching the enamel surface in a relatively short time forming a surface while forming a surface with increased roughness that enables micromechanical bonding of the adhesive on enamel.
- Optimal wetting and film-forming behaviour on the tooth surface and the capability of penetrating for example into dentinal tubules.

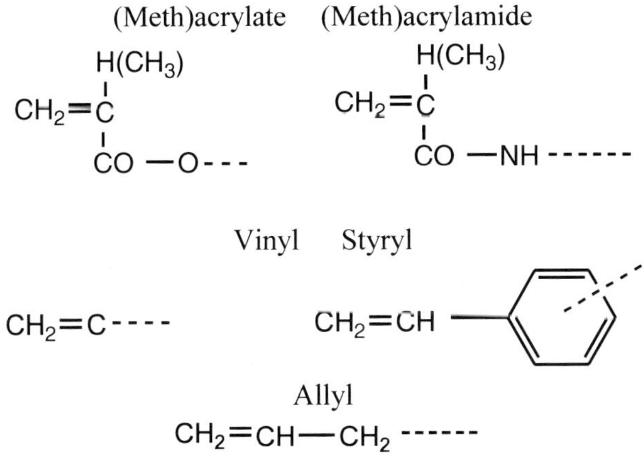

Figure 3.26. Polymerizable groups in monomers for adhesives.

- Fast ionic or covalent interaction with components of the dental hard tissue, e.g. the formation of low soluble calcium salts or formation of covalent bonds with collagen.

To achieve these specific requirements a great number of acidic monomers with the potential for generating a self-etching enamel-dentin adhesive have been described in the literature. In general these self-etching adhesive monomers are bifunctional molecules containing at least the following components: first a polymerizable group P, which can react both with the other monomers of the adhesive and the restorative material by copolymerization, second an acid adhesive group AD capable of both etching the dental hard tissues and interacting with the tooth substance and finally a spacer group designed to influence, e.g. the solubility, flexibility and wetting properties of the adhesive monomer (Figure 3.27) [88,95].

Suitable adhesive groups are acidic groups (Figure 3.28) in particular phosphoric acid, phosphonic acid which form stronger acids than the corresponiding carboxylic acids. The general potential of the acidic monomers to etch e.g. enamel largely depends on the acidity of the monomers that increase in the following order: carboxylic acids<phosphonic acids<acid phosphates<sulfonic acid. However, the application of polymerizable sulfonic acids in present self etching adhesive monomers should not only exhibit appropriate etching properties, but also meet the full set of requirements [88,95].

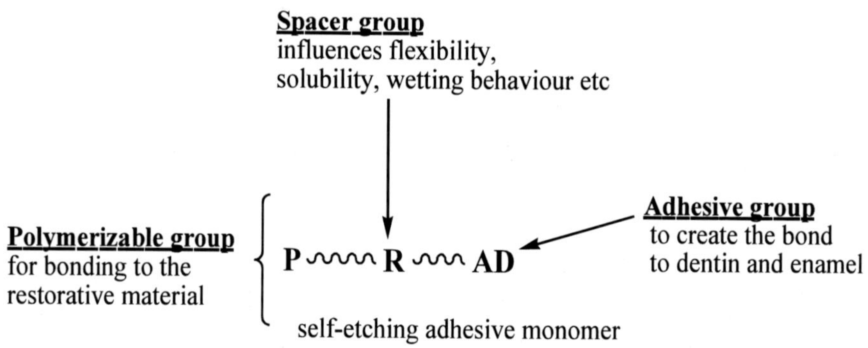

Figure 3.27. General structure of a self-etching adhesive monomer.

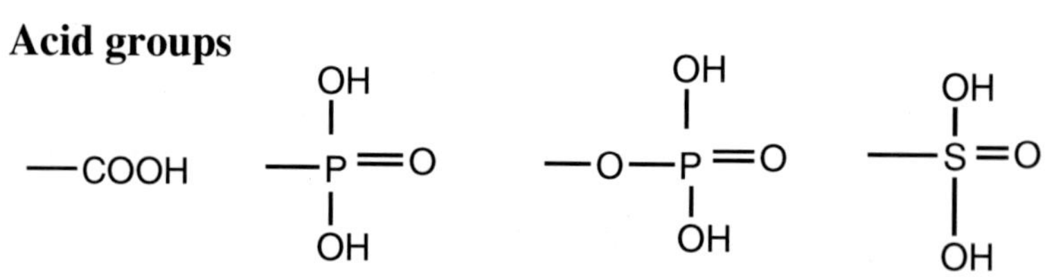

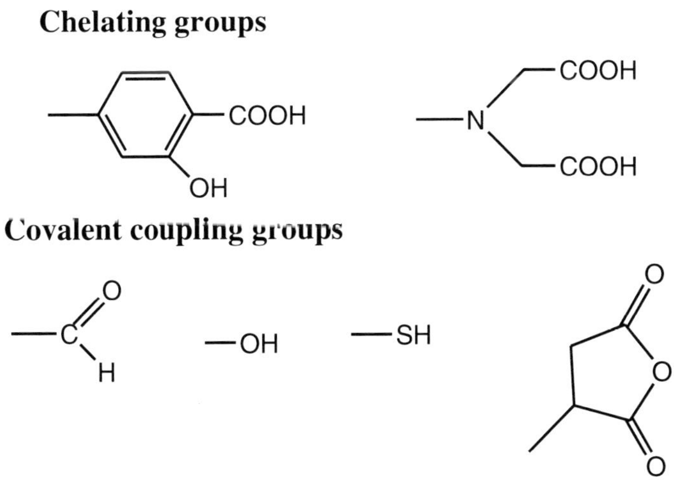

Figure 3.28. Adhesive groups AD enable chemical adhesion to enamel or dentin.

The chemical adhesion of monomers on the hard tissue of a natural tooth can be realized by the formation of primary chemical bonds, such as covalent or ionic bonds generated by the reaction of suitable adhesive groups with components of the dental hard tissue. As a consequence, ionic bonds are formed by the acidic groups reacting with the main inorganic component of the dental hard tissue, which is hydroxyapatite. In addition chelating groups which we can find, for example, in salicylic acid or aminodiacetic acids (Figure 3.29) enable the formation of coordinate linkages to the calcium ions of enamel or dentin. As dentinal collagen contains reactive groups, which are amino or hydroxyl groups in particular, the reaction of dentin with e.g. aldehyde (-CHO) or anhydride groups (-COOCO-) may establish covalent bonds with the collagen fibers, if conditions are mild. Moreover, secondary valence forces, such as attraction forces of molecular (Van der Waals forces) and induced dipoles (London dispersion forces) or attraction forces caused by the formation of hydrogen bridges or charge-transferinteractions may additionally contribute to the adhesion (physical adhesion) [88,95].

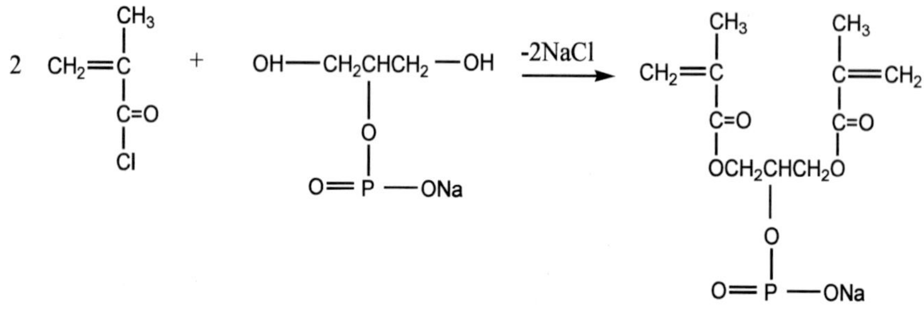

Figure 3.29. Reaction of glycerol 2-phosphate with methacryloyl chloride for the preparation of GDMP.

3.3.1. Adhesion Monomers in Commercial Self-etching Enamel-dentin Adhesives

3.3.1.1. Phosporous Containing Monomers [87,88,95,98]

The glycerol dimethacrylate ester of phosphoric acid (GDMP) was one of the first chemical compoundsto be investigated in an effort to improve the bonding to human dentine. It was prepared by the reaction of the disodium salt of glycerol 2-phosphate with methacryloyl chloride (Figure 3.29).

In general phosphorous-containing monomers are capable of etching enamel and dentine. Furthermore these monomers promote monomer diffusion into the acid-conditioned and underlying intact dentin. Therefore, various methacryloxyalkyl groups containing hydrogen (A) or dihydrogen phosphates (B) or diphosphates (C) (Figure 3.30) have been described in numerous patents [99-101].One of the first acidic methacrylate phosphates applied to improve the bond to dentin was the reaction product of phosphorous oxychloride with Bis-GMA [102]. Further examples of monomers that are used in practice, such as methacryloyloxyethylphenyl hydrogen phosphate (MEP-P), methacryloyloxydecyl hydrogen phosphate (MDP) methacryloyl oxypropyl dihydrogen phosphate (MPP) methacryloyloxyethyl dihydrogen phosphate (MEP) and dipentaerythrolpentaacryloyl dihydrogen phosphate (Penta-P) are summarized in Figure 3.31. These polymerizable strong acidic monomers enable the preparation of self-etching adhesives. Self-etching adhesives of this type are mostly used as a water-based solution of the polymerizable acidic phosphates. In the case of all the methacrylates phosphates shown in Figure 3.32 hydrolysis of the methacrylate ester bond will take place in the presence of water and is catalyzed by hydrogen ions of the phosphoric acid group. Moszner, Salz et al. [103] found that in the case of MEP both the hydrolysis of the methacrylate and phosphate ester bond occurs under formation of both methacrylic acid (MMA) and 2-hydroxyethyl methacrylate (HEMA) which is shown in Figure 3.32. In general the hydrolytic stability of phosphoric acid esters increases in the following order: trialkyl phosphate < dialkyl hydrogen phosphate < monoalkyl dihydrogen phosphate. Therefore, hydrolysis of the phosphate ester bond in the monoester MEP was not expected. Furthermore they found that in the case of longer alkylene spacers for example MDP the phosphate ester bond is more stable. Nevertheless, aqueous solutions of MDP are also not stable in storage at room temperature and have to be stored in a refrigerator.

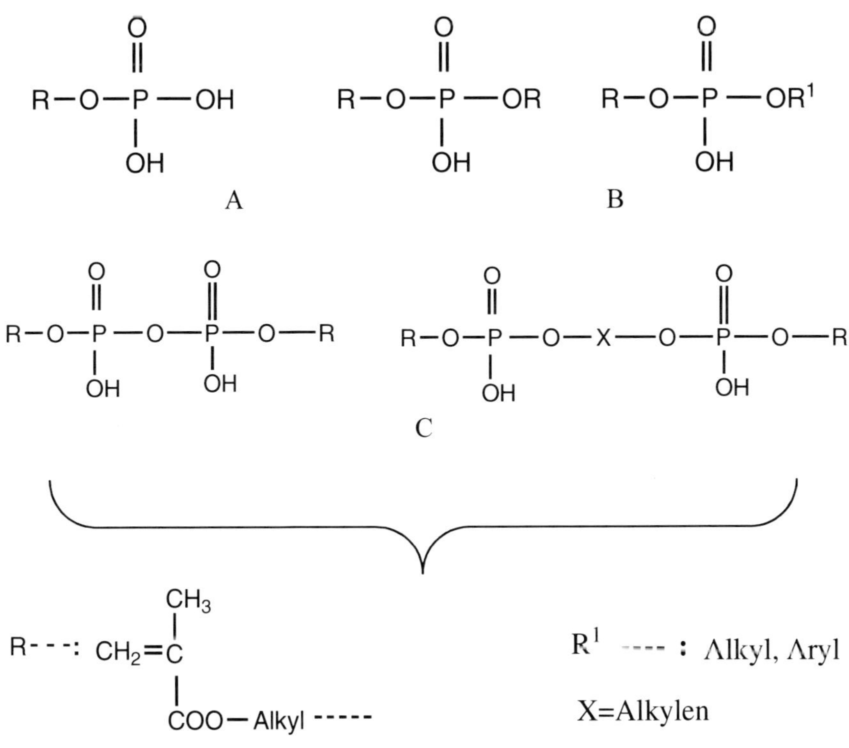

Figure 3.30. General formulas of methacryloyloxyalkyl hydrogen phosphates or diphosphates [88].

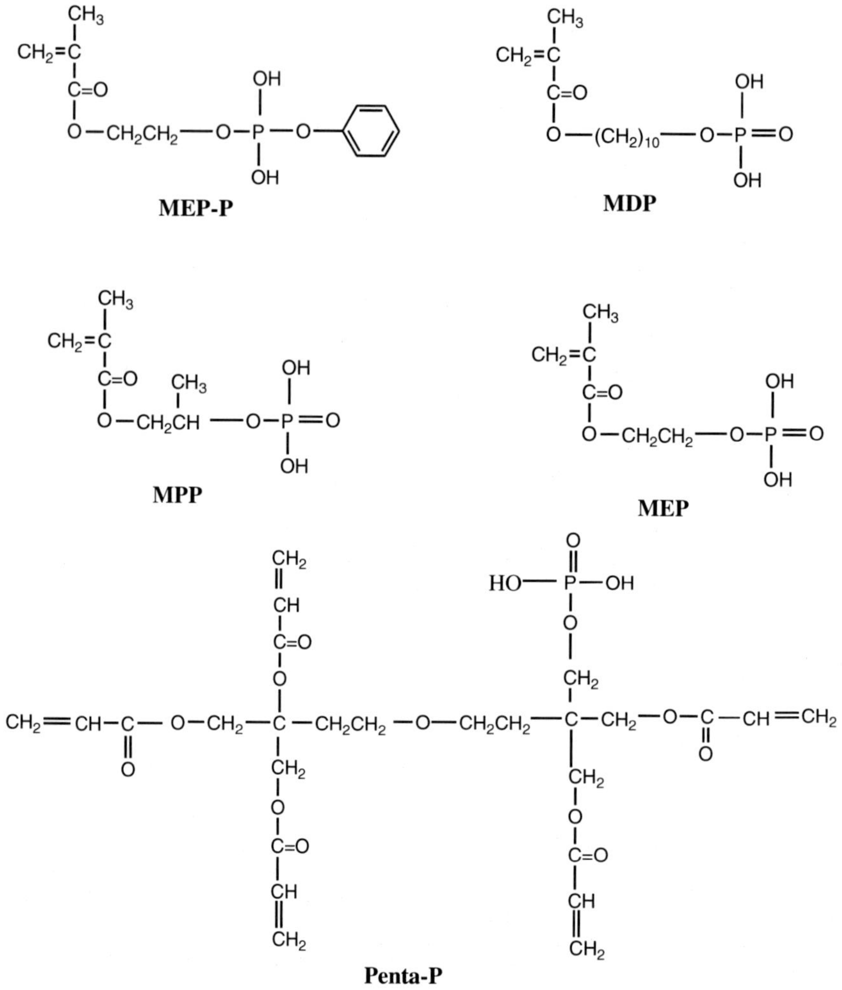

Figure 3.31. Examples of polymerizable acidic phosphates used in dental adhesives [87,88,95].

The problem of the hydrolytical instability of the methacrylate phosphates can be solved by applying monomers that contain more hydrolytically stable bonds between the polymerizable group and the strongly acidic phosphorous group. Phosphonates may be used for this purpose. Anbar et al. showed that vinylphoshonic acid (VPA) and 4-vinylbenzylphosphonic acid (VBPA) (Figure 3.33) or corresponding copolymers can improve the adhesion of filling composites on etched enamel and decrease the adsorption of proteins on enamel [104-106]. Unfortunately, VPA and VBPA are less reactive than methacrylates in free-radical polymerization. In this context Moszner et al. were able to prepare some new *a*crylic *e*ther *p*hosphonic *a*cids (AEPA) with improved hydrolytic stability and reactivity in the free-radical polymerization. In these acids the polymerizable methacrylate group and the strong acidic phosphorous group are connected through a hydrolytically stable ether group (Figure 3.34) [92,103, 107-109].

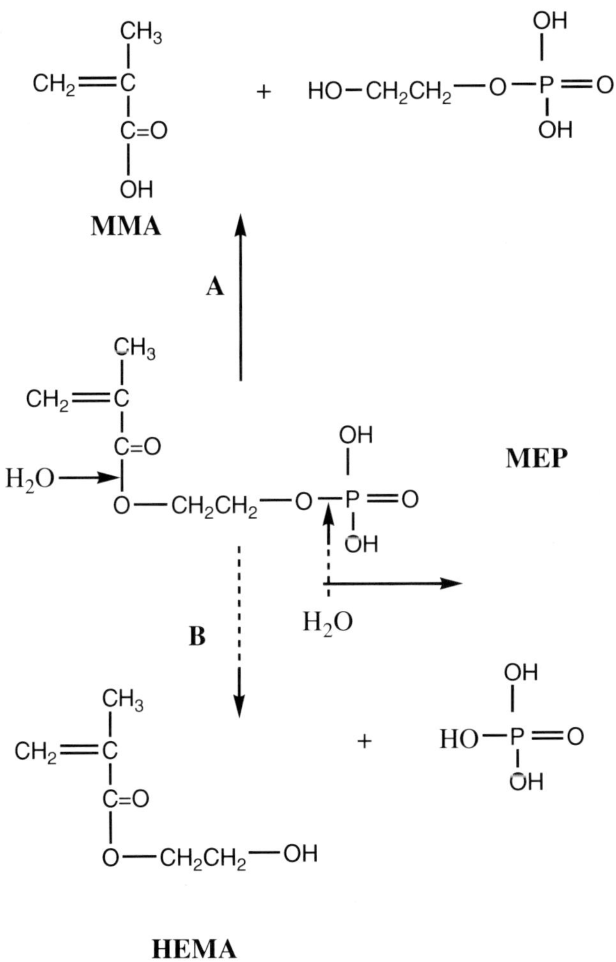

Figure 3.32. Hydrolysis of MEP in the presence of water.

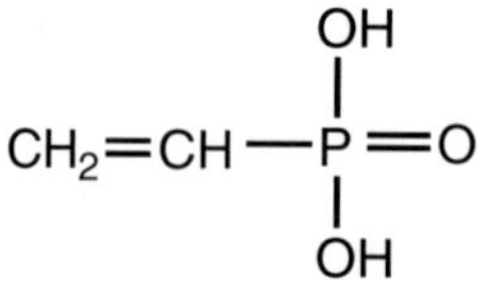

VPA

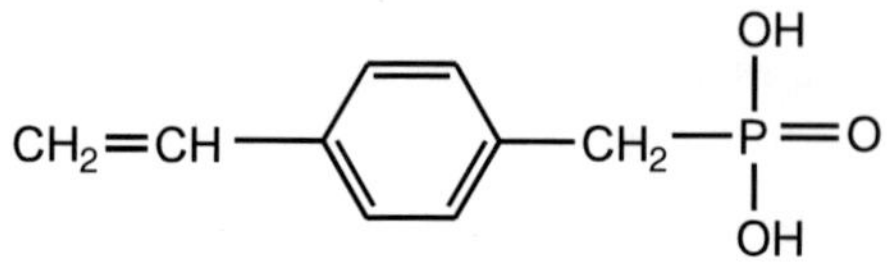

VBPA

Figure 3.33. Structure of the monomeric phosphonic acids VPA and VBPA.

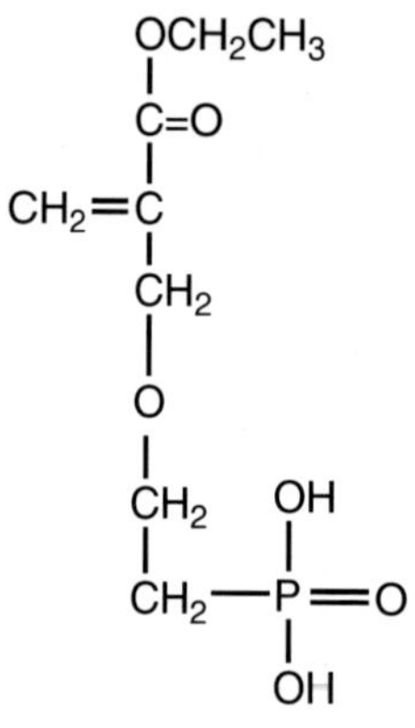

EAEPA

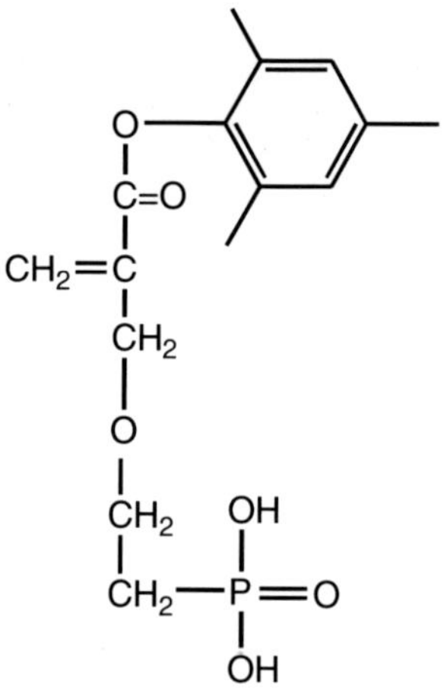

MAEPA

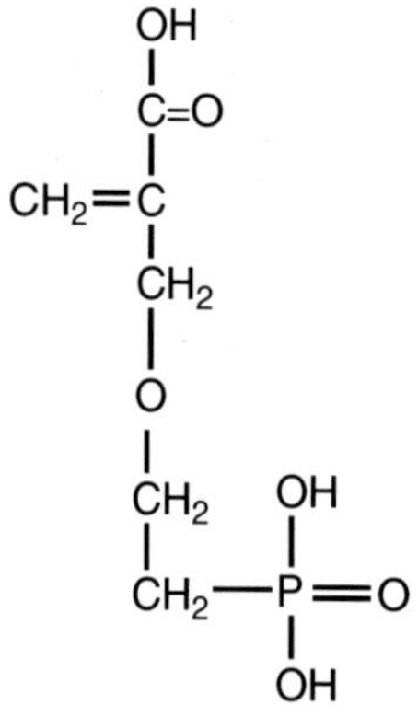

CAEPA

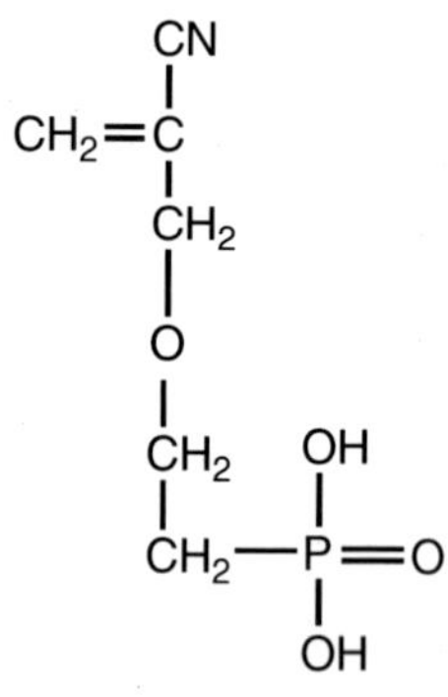

NAEPA

Figure 3.34. Structure of various acrylic ether phosphonic acids (AEPA).

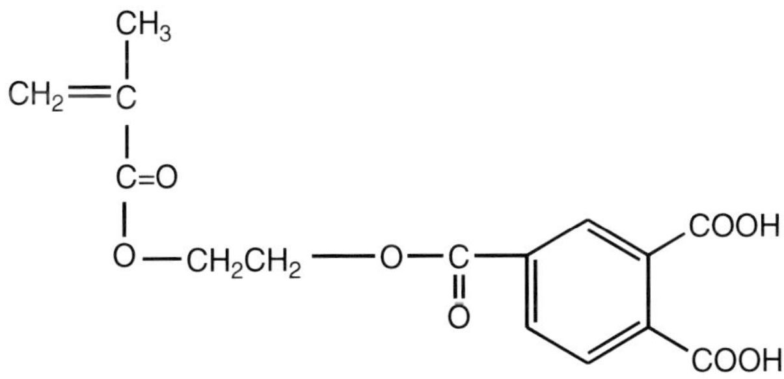

4-MET

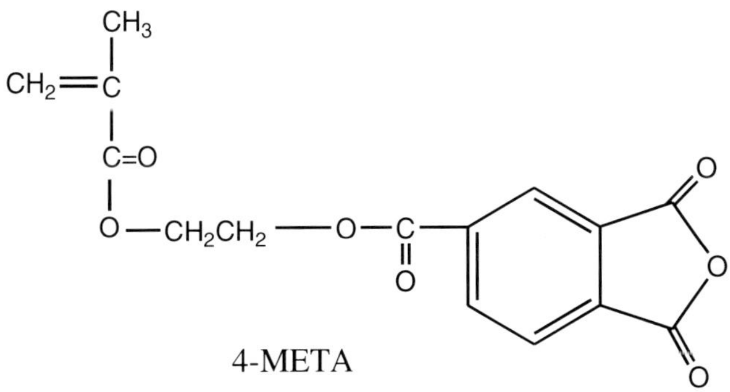

4-META

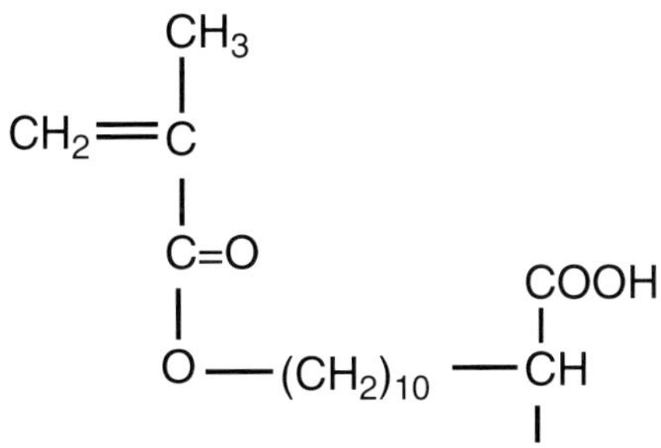

MAC-10

Figure 3.35. Structure of self-etching polymerizable carboxylic acids.

Due to their acidity the monomers are able to etch enamel or dentin. The etch pattern produced with the polymerizable phosphonic acids is similar to that generated by commercial etching gels based on 35 wt% phosphoric acid. Among the prepared monomers, EAEPA (ethyl 2-[4-(dihydroxyphosphoryl)-

2-oxabutyl]acrylate and MAEPA (2,4,6-trimethyl phenyl 2-[4-(dihydroxyphosphoryl)-2-oxabutyl]acrylate featured the best dentin adhesive properties; whereas the corresponding carboxylic acid group containing phosphonic acid CAEPA (2-[4-dihydroxy dihydroxyphosphoryl)-2-oxabutyl]acrylic acid) or the nitrile derivative NAEPA (2-[4-dihydroxy dihydroxyphosphoryl)-2-oxabutyl]acrylonitrile showed significantly less adhesion action.

3.3.1.2. Polymerizable Carboxylic Acids

The use of free-radically polymerizable unsaturated carboxylic acids in self-etching primers is restricted to only a few compounds such as the 4-methacryloyloxyethyl trimellitic acid (4-MET), 4-methacryloyloxyethyl trimellitate anhydride (4-META) and 10-methacryloyloxydecyl malonic acid (MAC-10) (Figure 3.35). Aqueous solutions of these polymerizable unsaturated carboxylic acids show a pH value below 2.0 as well and as consequence enable the surface of enamel and dentine to be etched [88].

3.3.2. Monofunctional and Crosslinking Monomers in Commercial Adhesives

Hydrophilic monomethacrylates are used as comonomers in self-etching enamel-dentin adhesives. Among the monomethacrylates HEMA is the most frequently applied monomer, while similar monomers, such as 2-hydroxy-propyl methacrylate (HPMA) or 2-hydroxy-3-phenoxy-propyl methacrylate (HPPMA) are rarely employed (Figure 3.36). HEMA is a water-soluble, low-viscosity monomer that improves the miscibility and solubility of the polar and non-polar adhesive components and the wetting behaviour of the liquid adhesive on dental hard tissue. In addition, it is well-known that HEMA may stabilize the collagen fibril network and improve the dentinal permeability and monomer diffusion [87,88]. However, HEMA is not hydrolytically stable under acidic aqueous conditions and forms associates in concentrated solutions, which promote its hydrolysis [110]. Furthermore it has to be considered that a high content of mono-functional monomers in the adhesive impair its polymerization rate. This may lead to a significant lower density of cross-linkage in the polymerized adhesive layer, which may result in weakened adhesive bonds, in particular, after storage and swelling in water.

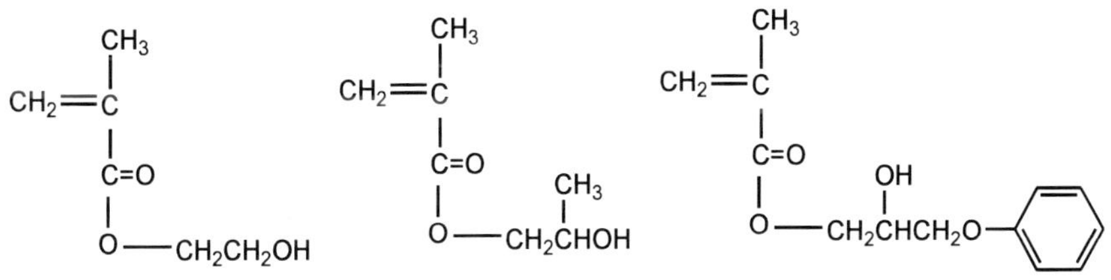

HEMA HPMA HPPMA

Figure 3.36. OH-group containing methacrylates used in dentine adhesives.

Hydrophilic cross-linking dimethacrylates are used in enamel-dentin adhesives to generate the formation of the polymer network, which leads to a number of favourable effects. Firstly the there is a strong increase in the polymerization rate because of the gel effect; secondly the mechanical properties of a polymer network are improved compared to linear polymers; and thirdly the formed the crosslinked layer is not water soluble and the degree of swelling decreases with increasing polymer network density. The dimethacrylates demonstrate different properties, such as viscosity, polarity, water solubility, polymerization shrinkage, film formation behaviour and reactivity. The most popular cross-linking dimethacrylates used in enamel-dentin adhesives are 2,2-bis[4-(2-hydroxy-3-methacryloyloxypropyl)-phenyl]propane (Bis-GMA), 1,6-bis-[2-methacryloyloxyethoxy-carbonylamino]-2,4,4-trimethylhexane (UDMA), glycerol dimethacrylate (GDMA) and triethylene glycol dimethacrylate (TEGDMA) (Figure 3.37). Bis-GMA shows a high reactivity in the free radical polymerization. However the viscosity is also vert high and the water solubility is low. In contrast to this, TEGDMA and GDMA are dimethacrylates featuring low viscosity and improved solubility in water. Unfortunately, all these dimethacrylates are not hydrolytically stable in acid aqueous acidic solutions and degrade under formation of corresponding diols and methacrylic acid [87,88].

TEGDMA and GDMA undergo rapid hydrolysis under acidic aqueous conditions. Therefore, they cannot be used for the preparation of water based single-bottle adhesives that remain stable if stored room temperature. It is well know that carbamides are more hydrolytically stable than esters because their carbonyl group exhibits a lower reactivity [88].Thus it can be expected that difunctional acryl- or methacrylamides exhibit enhanced hydrolytic stability compared to dimethacrylates. N,N' –ethylenebisacrylamide or N,N' –methylenebisacrylamide are commercially available and used as cross-linking agents for the preparation of poly(acrylamide) gels. However, these are solids and they feature a water solubility of less than 5%. Moreover they are practically insoluble in ethanol or aceton. Moszner et al. prepared three new bis(acrylamide)s (Figure 3.39) which are liquids and completely soluble in water and ethanol and show an improved hydrolytic stability [111]. These three bis(acrylamide)s are the N,N' –dimethyl-1,3-bis(acrylamido)-hexane (DMBAAH) the N,N' –dimethyl-1,3-bis(acrylamido)-propane (DMBAAP) and N,N' –diethyl-1,3-bis(acrylamido) propane (DEBAAP) (Figure 3.38). The water soluble bis(acrylamide)s show a similar reactivity with the cross-linking dimethacrylates as e.g. GDMA. Bis(methacrylamide)s are less reactive than the corresponding bis(acrylamide)s. In contrast to the GDMA, the water soluble bis(acrylamide)s as e.g. DEBAAP feature a significantly higher hydrolytic stability [88].

Analogous to the dimethacrylates, the monofunctional monomers and HEMA in particular also have to be substituted in water based single-bottle self etching enamel-dentin adhesives with appropriate monomers that exhibit enhanced hydrolytic stability as in the case e.g. (meth)acrylamides. HEMA substitutes are for example-methylolacrylamide (HMAM) or N-methylolmethacrylamide (HMMAM) (Figure 3.39) which are more effective in conjunction with suitable dentin primers than HEMA [112]. However it is reported that N-methylol compounds are degradable under formation of formaldehyde which is a toxicological risk. Therefore, monomers with a longer spacer between the OH group and the polymerizable (meth)acrylamide group would be advantageous [113]. Moszner et al. found that N-(2-hydroxyethyl)-methacrylamide (HEMAM) and N-methyl-N-(2-hydroxyethyl-acrylamide (MHEAM) feature improved hydrolytic stability and very low cytotoxicity [114]. They are therefore suitable to substitute HEMA in water based single-bottle self-etching enamel-dentin adhesives containing new strongly acidic adhesive monomers.

Finally some (meth) acrylamides were studied to be used as monomers for enamel and dentin adhesives. Examples for these are: N-methacryloyl-1-aminosalicylic acid (MASA) [115], N-acryloyl aspartic acid (NAASP) [116,117] and N-methacrylyoyl glycine (NMGLY) (Figure 3.40) [93]. The study of NMGLY showed that its hydrolytic stability was higher than that of HEMA.

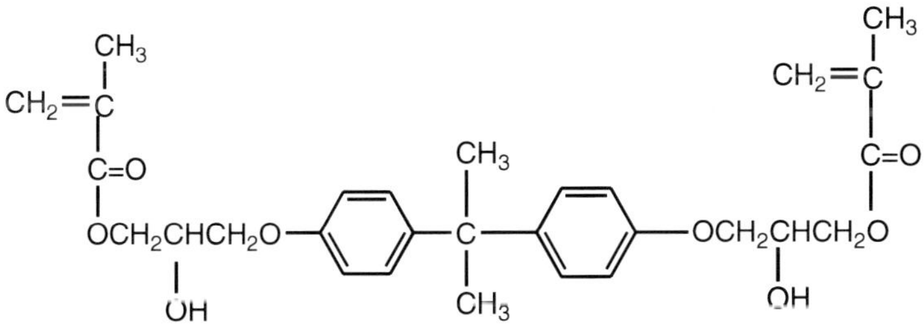

Bis-GMA

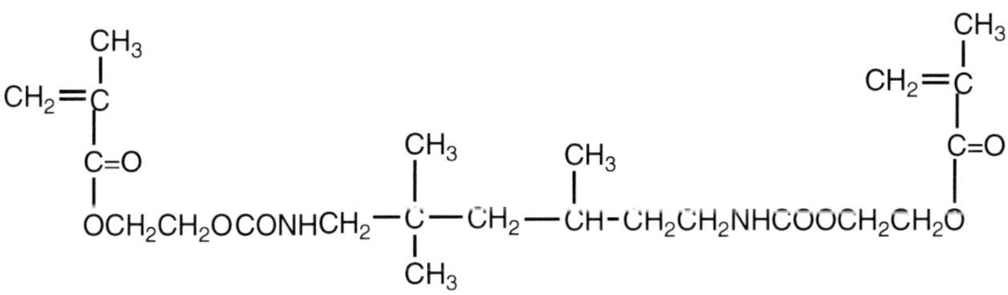

UDMA

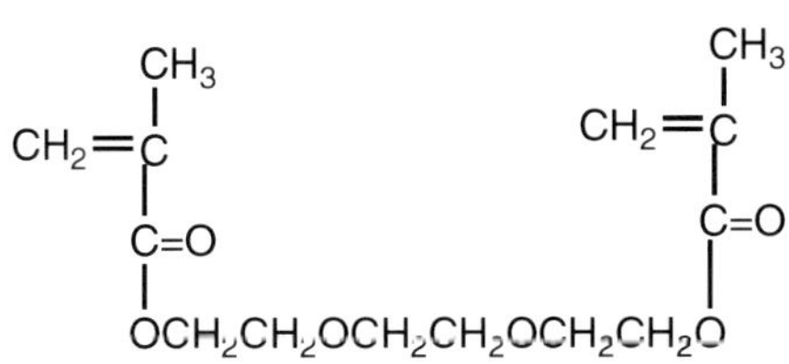

TEGDMA

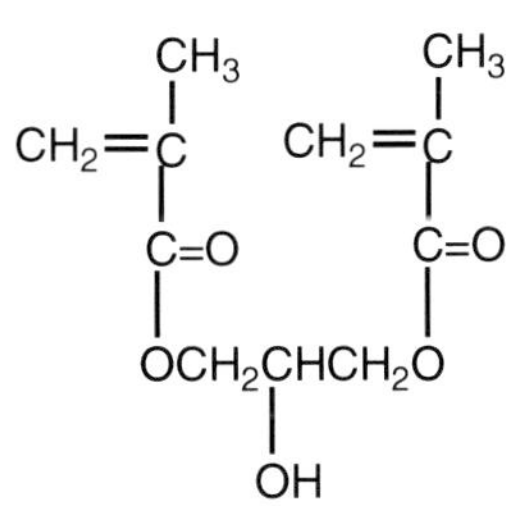

GDMA

Figure 3.37. Cross-linking dimethacrylates used in dentin adhesives.

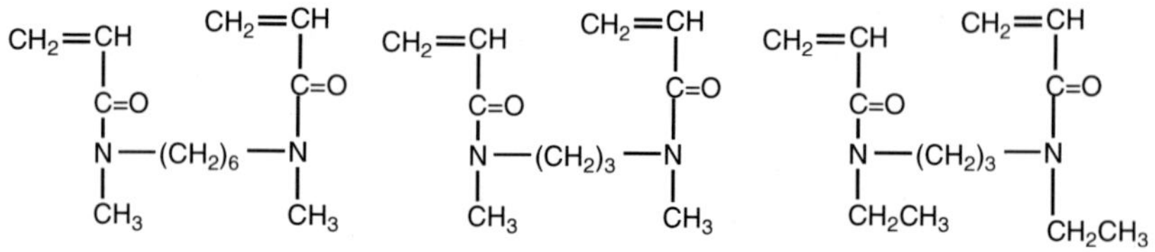

DMBAAH DMBAAP DEBAAP

Figure 3.38. Bis(acrylamide)s with improved hydrolytic stability.

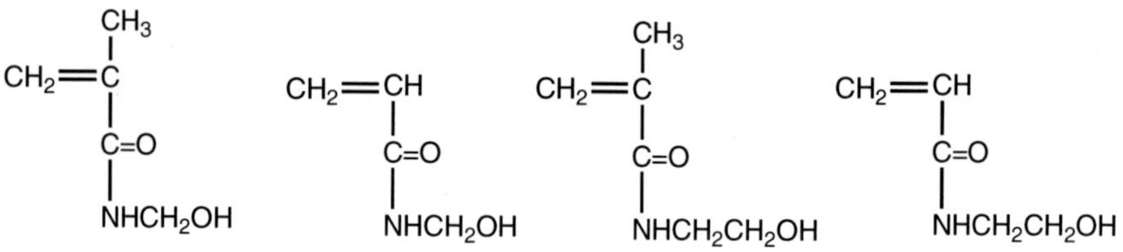

HMAM HMMAM HEMAM MHEAM

Figure 3.39. Substitutes of HEMA with improved hydrolytic stability.

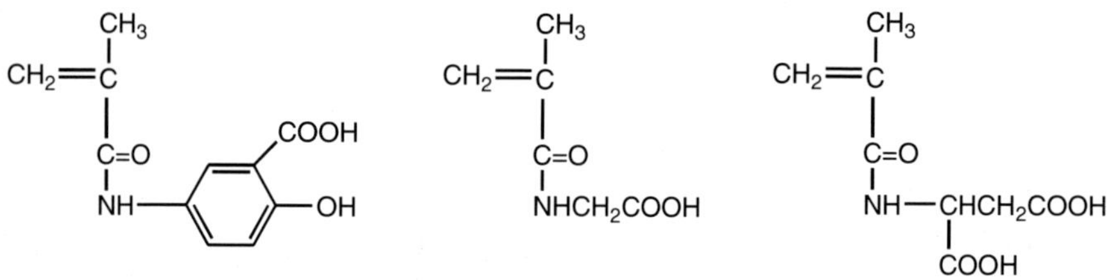

MASA NMGLY NAASP

Figure 3.40. (Meth) acrylamides containing –COOH groups.

3.3.3. Initiator Systems for Self-etching Adhesives

The monomers in dental adhesives are polymerized thanks to a free radical polymerization. In order to set off this reaction small amounts of initiator are required which will be consumed during the polymerization reaction. Initiators are generally molecules that possess atomic bonds with low dissociation energy that will form radicals under certain conditions. These radicals will set off the free-radical polymerization [89]. Radicals can be produced by a variety of photochemical or redox methods. In the first case photo-activated initiators are used and in the second case redox initiators. Photo-initiators absorb electromagnetic energy, while redox initiators need admixture of another component. The choice between photo-initiation and redox initiation depends on the purpose of the adhesive system. The main advantage of photo-initiation is the easy control of the onset of polymerization. However, whenever radiation is hampered to reach the adhesive redox initiation is the better choice. Generally adhesives devised to bond composite fillings utilize photo-initiators, whereas polymer-based cements usually rely on redox initiation. When both photo-initiators and redox initiators are added the adhesive is said to be "dual-curing". The aim of this double setting mechanism is mainly to boost the polymerization and consequently to achieve a higher degree of conversion, especially at areas remote or hidden from the light source. The amount of initiator added to adhesive systems depends on the type of initiator and on the adhesion system, but is usually very small in the range of 0.1-1wt%.

An intrinsic problem of self-etching enamel-dentin adhesives is the acid-base reaction of the acidic monomers with amines often used in the initiator systems, such as the camphorquinone/amine system in visible light curing adhesives or the peroxide/amine redox system. In both cases, the concentration of amine and therefore, also of the formed amine radical, which is responsible for the initiation of polymerization, decreases. The acid-base reaction results in an equilibrium between the protonized and unprotonized form of the amine and the acid (Figure 3.41).Therefore the amine concentration needs to be exactly adjusted to the concentration of acid in self-etching systems [88].

Adhesives cured by a redox initiator system are even more sensitive due to the thicker oxygen inhibition layers. This has resulted in alternatively using less sensitive redox initiators containing reductants such as barbituric acid [118] ascorbic acid [119] sulfinic acid [120] or combinations of them with amine/peroxide systems [94, 123].

In the case of photoinitiators, carbonyl compounds which absorb light in the wavelength 400-500 nm, undergo Norrish type I photo-fragmentation and do not require amine accelerators, are needed. Examples of such compounds are benzoin esters, benzophenone and acylphosphine oxides. The latter were introduced on the market some years ago as a new class of of a-cleavage photoinitiators [39].The absorption characteristics of acylphosphine oxides differ from most other photoinitiators of the a-cleavage type in that they feature enhanced absorption in the near UV/Vis range. This is very important for their use in dental materials, e.g. dental adhesives. The chemical structure of an acylphosphine oxide is shown in Figure 3.42. A disadvantage of acylphosphine oxides is that they are not compatible with most of the new dental LED polymerization light units and that acylphosphine oxides are prone to undergoing solvolytic cleavage of the carbon-phosphorous bond in the presence of nucleophilic compounds such as water or alcohols [122].

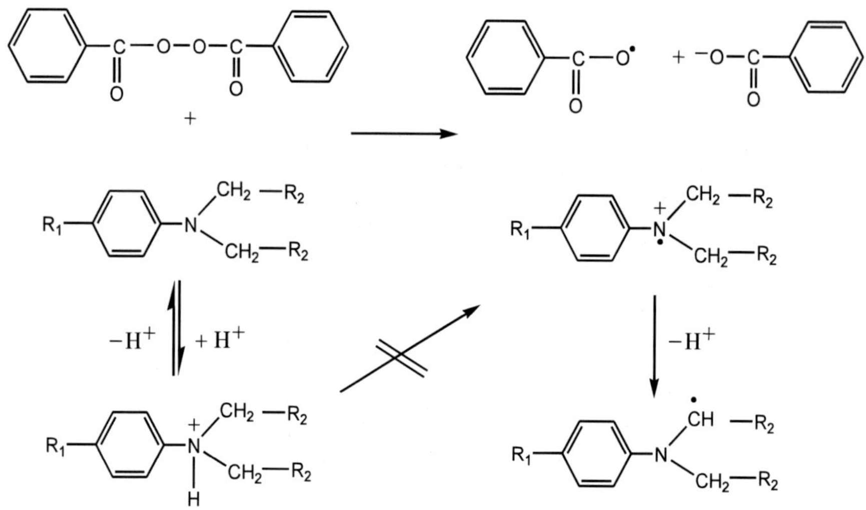

Figure 3.41. Acid-base reaction of an amine/peroxide redox initiator system for radical polymerization.

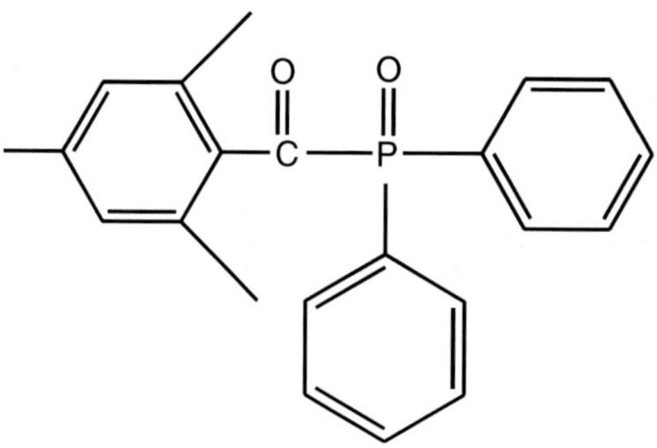

Figure 3.42. Chemical structure of acylphosphine oxide.

3.3.4. Solvent

Solvents are substances that are capable of dissolving one or more other substances.When a solvent dissolves a solid or a liquid the molecules become separated from each other and the spaces between them become occupied by solvent molecules. The energy required to break the bonds between the solute particles is supplied by the formation of bonds between the solute particles and the solvent molecules; the old intermolecular forces are replaced by new ones. The solubility characteristics of molecules are determined chiefly by their polarity. Non-polar or weakly polar compounds dissolve in non-polar or weakly polar solvents; highly polar compounds dissolve in highly polar solvents ("like dissolves like"). The polarity of solvents is determined by both the dipole moment and the dielectric constant. Solvents have been classified into three categories according to their polarity: polar protic, polar aprotic, and apolar solvents. Polar protic solvents consist of a hydroxyl-group that can form strong hydrogen bonds, such as water and ethanol. Polar aprotic solvents do not have the required hydroxyl groups to form hydrogen bonds but do have a large dipole moment. They usually also contain a keton group, such as acetone. Apolar solvents have both a low dielectric constant and dipole moment. The polarity of a solvent is also important to predict the self life of adhesives, as apolar solvents will more easily pass through traditional polyethylene packaging. In adhesives, water, ethanol and acetone are the most commonly used solvents. The use of these solvents in adhesives must be explained by their inexpensiveness, their wide availability and their good biocompatibility. Most other typical solvents are toxic [98].

3.3.5. Filler

Adhesives on the contrary to polymer composites not always contain filler particles. There are adhesives which contain filler particles and are characterized as "filled" and there are also adhesives which do not contain filler particles and characterized as "unfilled". Adhesives for bonding direct restorations to tooth tissue traditionally did not contain filler particles [88,98].

3.4. Literature

[1] Graig R.G. *Restorative dental materials;* Editor Graig R.G. and Ward M.L. 10th ed. Mosby: St. Louis, pp. 209-243.

[2] Peutzfeldt A. Resin composites in dentistry: the monomer systems. *Eur J Oral Sci.* 1997; 105: 97-116.

[3] Kim J.W.; Kim L.U.; and Kim C.K. Size control of silica nanoparticles and their surface treatment for fabrication of dental nanocomposites. *Biomacromolecules* 2007, 8, 215-222.

[4] Moszner N. New Monomers for Dental Application. *Macromol. Symp.* 2004, 217, 63-75.

[5] *Moszner Norbert and Ulrich Salz in Composites for dental restorat*ives; Editor, Shalaby W. Shalaby and Ulrich Salz. Taylor and Francis Group, 6000 Broken Sound Parkway NW, Suite 300, Boca Raton, FL 33487-2742, 2007; pp 14-58.

[6] Moszner Norbert and Simone Klapdohr. Nanotechnology for dental composites. *Int. J. of Nanotechnology,* 2004, Vol. 1, pp 130-156.

[7] Sideridou I.D., Tserki V., Papanastasiou G. Effect of chemical structure on degree of conversion in light-cured dimethacrylate-based dental resins. *Biomaterials* 2002, 23, 1819-1829.

[8] Sideridou I.D.; Achilias D.S.; Karava Olga. Reactivity of benzoyl peroxide/amine system as an initiator for the free radical polymerization of dental and orthopaedic dimethacrylate monomers: effect of the amine and monomer chemical structure. *Macromolecules* 2006, 39, 2072-2080.

[9] Achilias D.S.; Sideridou I.D. Kinetics of the benzoyl peroxide/amine initiated free radical polymerization of dental dimethacrylate monomers: experimental studies and mathematical modeling for TEGDMA and Bis-EMA. *Macromolecules* 2004, 37, 4254-4265.

[10] Achilias D.S.; Sideridou I.D. Study of the effect of two BPO/amine initiation systems on the free radical polymerization of MMA used in dental resins and bone cements. *J. Macromol, Sci., Part A: Pure Appl. Chem.* 2002, A39, 1435-1450.

[11] Sideridou I.D.; Achilias D.S.; Kostidou N.C. Copolymerization kinetics of dental dimethacrylates resins initiated by a benzoyl peroxide/amine redox system. *J. Appl. Polym. Sci.* 2008, 199: 515-524.

[12] Vazquez B.; Elvira C.; Roman J.S.; Levenfeld B. Reactivity of a polymerizable amine activator in the free radical copolymerization with methyl methacrylate and surface properties of copolymers. *Polymer* 1997, 38, 4365-4372.

[13] Dietliker K. In radiation curing in polymer science and technology; Editor Fouassier, J.P. and Rabek J.E. *Elsevier Applied Science*. London and New York. 1993, pp.188

[14] Ferracane J.L. Current Trends in Dental Composites. *Crit Rev Oral Biol Med* 1995, 6 (4), 302-318.

[15] Simone Klapdohr and Norbert Moszner; New inorganic Components for Dental Filling Composites. *Monatshefte fur Chemie* 136, 21-45, 2005.

[16] Morbert Norbert and Salz Ulrich; In *polymers for dental and orthopedic applications;* Editors Shalaby W. Shalaby and Ulrich Salz. CRC Press Taylor and Francis Group, Boca Raton, London, New York. 2007, pp. 15-5.

[17] Sideridou I., Achilias D.S., Kyrikou E. Thermal expansion characteristics of light-cured dental resins and resin composites. *Biomaterials* 25 (2004) 3087-3097.

[18] Richard van Noort. *Introduction to Dental Materials.* Mosby 2nd ed, London, 2006.

[19] Charlon G. D. *Resin composites.* https--decs.nhgl.med.navy.mil-DMNOTES-composites.pdf.

[20] Geraldı S.; Perdigao J. Microleakage of a new restorative system in posterior teeth. *J. Dent Res.* 2003; 81: 1276.

[21] Meyer G.R.; Ernst C.P.; Willershausen B. Determination of polymerization stress of conventional and new "clustered" microfill-composites in comparison with hybrid composites. *J. Dent Res* 2003; 81: 921.

[22] Matinlinna J.P. An introduction to silanes and their clinical applications in dentistry. *Int J Prosthodont* 2004, 17: 155-164.

[23] Antonucci J.M.; Dickens S.H.; Fowler B.O.; Xu H.H.K.; McDonough W. G. Chemistry of silanes: interfaces in dental polymers and composites. *J. Res. Natl. Inst. Stand. Technol.* 110, 541-558 (2005).

[24] Karabela, M.; Siderıdou, I. Effect of the structure of silane coupling agent on sorption characteristics of solvents by dental resin-nanocomposites. *Dental Materials.* 24, 1631-1639 (2008).

[25] Sideridou, I.D.; Karabela, M.M. Effect of the structure of silane-coupling agent on dynamic mechanical properties of dental resin-nanocomposites. *J Applied Polymer Science*, 110, 507-516 (2008).

[26] Plueddemann, E.P. *Silane Coupling Agents. Second Edition.* New York. Plenum Press. 1991.

[27] Chen, T.M.; Brauer, G.M. (1982). Solvent effects on bonding organo-silane to silica surfaces. *J Dent Res,* 61, 1439-1443.

[28] Venhoven, B.A.; de Gee, A.J. Werner, A.; and Davidson, C.L. (1994). Silane treatment of filler and composite bleding in a one-step procedure for dental restoratives. *Biomaterials* 15, 1152-1156.

[29] Wilson, K.S.; Zhang, K.; Antonucci, J.M. (2005). Systematic variation of interfacial phase reactivity in dental nanocomposites. *Biomaterials,* 26, 5095-103.

[30] Wilson, K.S.; Antonucci, J.M. (2006). Interphase structure-property relationship in thermoset dimethacrylate nanocomposites. *Dent Mater,* 22, 995-1001.

[31] Wilson, K.S.; Allen, A.J.; Washburn, N.R.; Antonucci, J.M. (2007). Interphase effects in dental nanocomposites investigated by small-angle neutron scattering. *J Biomed Mater Res,* 81A, 113-23.

[32] Söderholm, K.-J.M. and Shang, S.-W. (1993). Molecular orientation of silane at the surface of colloidal silica. *J Dent Res,* 72: 1050-1054.

[33] Miller, J.D.; Ishida, H. (1984). Quantitative monomolecular coverage of inorganic particulates by methacryl-functional silanes. *Surf Sci* , 148, 601-22.

[34] Kaas, R.L.; Kardos, J.L. (1971). The interaction of alkoxy silane coupling agents with silica surfaces. *Polymer Engineering and Science,* 11: 11-18.

[35] Jang, J.; Kim, S. (1996). Factors affecting diametral tensile strength of microfilled dental composites. *Polym J* , 28, 293-8.

[36] Nishiyama N, Katsuki H, Horie K, Asakura T. (1987). Adsorbed behavior of spin- labeled silane coupling agent on colloidal silica studied by electron spin resonance. *J Biomed Mater Res,* Part A 21, 1029-1038.

[37] Bauer, F.; Ernst, H.; Decker, U.; Findeisen, M.; Glasel, H-J.; Langguth, H.; Hartmann, E.; Mehnert, R.; Peuker, C. (2000). Preparation of scratch and abrasion resistant polymeric nanocomposites by monomer grafting onto nanoparticles,1. FTIR and multi-nuclear NMR spectroscopy to the characterization of methacryl grafting. *Macromol Chem Phys* 201, 2654-2659.

[38] Glasel, H-J.; Bauer, F.; Ernst, H.; Findeisen, M.; Findeisen, M.; Langguth, H.; Mehnert, R.; Schubert, R. (2000). Preparation of scratch and abrasion resistant polymeric nanocomposites by monomer grafting onto nanoparticles,2[a]. Characterization of radiation-cured polymeric nanocomposites. *Macromol Chem Phys,* 201, 2765-2770.

[39] Mathias, J.; Wannemacher, G. (1988). Basic characteristics and applications of aerosol. 30. The chemistry and Physics of the aerosol Surface. *J Colloid and Interface Science,* 125, 61-68.

[40] Liu, Q.; Ding, J.; Chambers, DE.; Debnath, S.; Wunder, SL.; Baran, GR. (2001). Filler-coupling agent-matrix interactions in silica/polymethylmethacrylate composites. *J Biomed Mater Res,* 57, 384-393.

[41] Antonucci, J.M.; McDonough, W.J.; Schutte, C.L.; Moon, C.K. (1995). Shear strength measurements of dental polymer/glass fiber interface via the microbond test. *Polymer Preprints,* 36, 821-822.

[42] McDonough, W.G.; Antonucci, J.M.; Dunkers, J.P. (1997). A study of dental adhesion by means of the microbond test. *Polymer Preprints*, 36 112-113.

[43] McDonough, W.G.; Antonucci, J.M.; Dunkers, J.P. (2001). Interfacial shear strengths of dental resin-glass fibersby the microbond test. *Dent Mater* 17, 492-498.

[44] Antonucci, J.M.; Stansbury, J.W.; Kim, S.I. (1995). Effect of a long-chain silane coupling agent on composite strength. *J Dent Res* 74, Abst No 461.

[45] Venz, S.; Antonucci, J.M. (1986). Silanization and modification of fillers for dental composites. *J Dent Res* 65, 191, Abstr. No. 191.

[46] Klapdohr, S.; Moszner, N. (2005). New Inorganic Components for Dental Filling Composites. *Monatshefte fur Chemie Chemical Monthly.* 136, 21-45.

[47] Plueddemann, EP.; Pape PG. (1985). The use of mixed silane coupling agents. In Preceedings, 40th Annual Conference, Reinforced Plastics/Composites Institute. *The Society of the Plastics Industry,* Inc., Session 17-F:1-4.

[48] Kurata, S.; Yamazaki, N. (1993). Effect of silane coupling agents with a bisfunctional hydrolyzable group. *Dent Mater J,* 12, 127-135.

[49] Craig, RG.; Dootz, ER. (1996). Effect of mixed silanes on the hydrolytic stability of composites. *J Oral Rehabil,* 23, 751-756.

[50] Nihei, T.; Kurata, S.; Kondo, Y.; Umemoto, K.; Yoshino, N.; Teranaka, T. (2002). Enhanced hydrolytic stability of dental composites by use of fluoroalkyltrimethoxysilanes. *J Dent Res* 81, 482-6.

[51] Matinlinna, J.P.; Lassila, L.V.J.; Vallittu, P.K. (2006). The effect of three silane coupling agents and their blends with a cross-linker silane on bonding a bis-GMA resin to silicatized titanium (a novel silane system). *Journal of Dentistry,* 34, 740-746.

[52] Matinlinna, J.P.; Lassila, L.V.J.; Vallittu, P.K. (2006). The effect of a novel silane blend system on resin bond strength to silica coated Ti substrate. *Journal of Dentistry* 34, 436-43.

[53] Nihei, T.; Dabanoglou, A.; Teranaka, T.; Kurata, S.; Ohashi, K.; Kondo, Y.; Yoshino, N.; Hickel, R.; Kunzelmann, K-H. (2008). Three-body wear resistance of the experimental composites containing filler treated with hydrophobic silane coupling agents. *Dent Mater* 24, 760-764.

[54] Matinlinna, J.P.; Lassila, L.V.J.; Kangasasniemi, I.; Vallittu, P.K. (2005). *Isocyanato- and Methacryloxysilanes Promote Bis-GMA Adhesion to Titanium.* 84, 360-364.

[55] Karabela, M.M.; Sideridou, ID. (2009). *Effect of the structure of silane-coupling agent on sorption characteristics of solvents by dental resin-nanocomposites.* Dent Mater, in press.

[56] Sideridou, ID.; Karabela, M.M. (2008). Effect of the Structure of Silane-Coupling Agent on Dynamic Mechanical Properties of Dental Resin-Nanocomposites. *J Appl Polym Sci* 110, 507–516.

[57] Combe E.D.; Burke F.J.T.; Douglas W.H.; *Dental Biomaterials.* Kluwer Academic Publishers, Boston, 1999, pp.239.

[58] Craig R.G.; Powers J.M.; Wataha J.C. *Dental Materials, Properties and Manipulation.* Mosby, Inc. 11830 Westline Industrial Drive, St. Louis, Missouri 64 146, 2000, Chapter 4, p. 57-76.

[59] Sideridou I.D.; Karabela M.M.; Micheliou C.N.; Karagiannidis P.G.; Logothetidis S. (2009). Physical Properties of a Hybrid and a nanohybrid dental light-cured resin composite. *Journal of Biomaterials Science* 20, 1831-1844.

[60] Sideridou I.; V. Tserki, G. Papanastasiou. (2003). Study of water sorption, solubility and modulus of elasticity of light-cured dimethacrylate-based dental resins. *Biomaterials,* 24, 655-665.

[61] Sideridou I.; Achilias D.S.; Spyroudi Ch.; Karabela M.(2004) Water sorption characteristics of light-cured dental resins and composites based on Bis-EMA/PCDMA. *Biomaterials,* 25, 367-376.

[62] Sideridou I.D.; Achilias D.S.; Karabela M.M. (2007). Sorption Kinetics of Ethanol/Water solution by dimethacrylate-based Dental Resins and Resin Composites. *J Biomed Mater Res Part B: Appl Biomater* 81B, 207-218.

[63] Sideridou I.D.; Papanastasiou G.E. (2008). Sorption of binary liquid mixtures in methacrylate-based biomaterials, simultaneous determination of the diffusion coefficients and the uptake fraction at equilibrium of the components of ethanol-water mixtures by a new iterative method. *J Appl Polym Sci* , 107, 1057-1066.

[64] Sideridou I.D.; Papanastasiou G.E. (2007).Water sorption kinetics in light- cured poly-HEMA and poly(HEMA-co-TEGDMA);

Determination of the self-diffusion coefficient by new iterative methods. *J Appl Polym Sci* , 106, 2380-2390.
[65] Sideridou I.D.; Karabela M.M.; Vouvoudi E.Ch.; Papanastasiou, G. (2008). Sorption and desorption parameters of water or ethanol in light-cured dental dimethacrylate resins. *J Applied Polymer Science,* 107, 463-475.
[66] Sideridou I.D.; Karabela M.M.; Vouvoudi E.Ch.(2008). Volumetric dimensional changes of dental light-cured dimethacrylate resins after sorption of water or ethanol. *Dental Materials,* 24; 1131-1136.
[67] Sideridou I.D.; Achilias D.S. (2005). Elution study of unreacted Bis-GMA, TEGDMA, UDMA, and Bis-EMA from light-cured dental resins and resin composites using HPLC. *J. Biomed Mater Res Part B: Appl Biomater,* 74B, 617-626.
[68] Sideridou I., Achilias D.S.; Kyrikou, E. (2004). Thermal expansion characteristics of light-cured dental resins and resin composites. *Biomaterials,* 25, 3087-3097.
[69] Geurtsen W. (1998). Substances released from dental resin composites and glass ionomer cements. *Eur J Oral Sci,* 106, 687-695.
[70] Schmalz G. (1998). The biocompatibility of non-amalgam dental filling materials. *Eur J Oral Sci,* 106, 696-706.
[71] Salz Ulrich In Ivoclar-Vivadent Report no.7, November 1992.
[72] Sideridou I.D.; Karabela M.M.; Bikiaris D.N. (2007) Aging studies of light-cured dimethacrylate-based dental resins and a resin composite in water or ethanol/water. *Dental Materials* 23, 1142-1149.
[73] Sideridou I.D.; Karabela M.M.; Vouvoudi E.Ch. (2008) Dynamic thermomechanical properties and sorption characteristics of two commercial light cured dental resin composites. *Dental Materials* 24, 737-743.
[74] Sideridou I.D.; Karabela M.M.; Spyroudi C.S. (2009). Dynamic mechanical analysis of a hybrid and a nanohybrid light-cured dental resi composite. *Journal of Biomaterials Science,* 20 (1797-1808).
[75] Ott G. In Ivoclar-Vivadent Report no.5, February 1990.
[76] http://www.animated-teeth.com/tooth_sealants/t1a_sealing_teeth.htm
[77] http://users.forthnet.gr/ath/abyss/dep1411.htm
[78] http://users.forthnet.gr/ath/abyss/dep1151.htm
[79] Buonocore, M.G. (1955). A simple method of increasing the adhesion of acrylic filling materials to enamel surfaces. *J Dent Res* 34, 849-53.
[80] Simonsen, R.J. (2004) Pit and Fissure Sealant: Then, now and next steps. *J Public Health Dentistry,* 64, 17-22.

[81] Tsuchitani, Y.; Wada, T. Pit and Fissure Sealants. In: Salamone JC, editor. *Polymeric Materials Encyclopedia.* New York. CRC Press, Inc; 1996; 1868-1870.

[82] Yamauchi, J.; Yamada, K.; Shibatani, K. (1980). *Adhesive compositions for the hard tissues of the human body.* U.S. Patent 4 182 035.

[83] Dart, E.C.; Nemcek, J.; (1975). Photopolymerizable composition. *Great Britain Patent* 1408265.

[84] Kadoma, Y. Masuhara, E. (1981) Controlled release of fluoride ions from methacryloyl fluoride-methyl methacrylate copolymers 1. Synthesis of methacryoyl fluoride and methyl methacrylate copolymers. *Makromol Chem,* 182, 273-277.

[85] Combe, E.C.; Burke, F.J.T; Douglas, W.H. *Dental Biomaterials.* Boston: Kluwer Academic Publishers; 1999.

[86] Van Meerbeek B.; Kanumilli, P.; De Munck, J.; Van Landuyt, K.; Lambrechets, P.; Peumans, M.(2005). "A randomized controlled study evaluating the effectiveness of a two-step self-etch adhesive with and without selective phosphoric-acid etching". *Dental Materials,* 21, 375-383.

[87] Moszner N.; Salz, U. (2007). Recent Developments of New Components for Dental Adhesives and Composites. *Macromolecular Materials and Engineering,* 292, 245-271.

[88] Moszner N.; Salz, U. Zimmermann, J. (2005) Chemical aspects of self-etching enamel-dentin adhesives: A systematic review. *Dental Materials*, 21, 895-910.

[89] Odian G. *Principles of Polymerization.* NY:Wiley Interscience. (2004).

[90] Peutzfeldt, A.(1997). Resin composites in dentistry; the monomer systems. *Eur J Oral Sci,* 105, 97-106

[91] Lee, T.Y.; Guymon, C.A.; Jonsson, E.S.; Hoyle, C.E. (2004). The effect of monomer structure on oxygen inhibition of (meth)acrylates photopolymerization. *Polymer,* 45, 6155-62.

[92] Salz, U.; Zimmermann, J.; Zeuner, F.; Moszner, N. (2005). Hydrolytic stability of self-etching adhesive systems. *J. Adhes Dent,* 7, 107-16.

[93] Nishiyama, N.; Suzuki, K.; Yoshida, H.; Teshima, H.; Nemoto, K. (2004). Hydrolytic stability of methacrylamide in acidic aqueous solution. *Biomaterials,* 25, 965-9.

[94] Salz, U.; Zimmermann, J.; Salzer, T. (2005). Self- etching adhesive cement systems. *J Adhes Dent,* 7, 7-17.

[95] Salz, U.; Moszner N. Enamel and Dentin Adhesion. In: Shalaby, S.W.; Salz, U. Editors. *Polymers for Dental and Orthopedic Applications.* NW: Taylor and Francis Group; 2007; p.106.

[96] Nishyama, N.; Suzuki, K.; Takahashi, K.; Nemoto, K. (2004). The p*K*a effects of the carboxylic acid in N-methacryloyl omega-amino acid on the demineralization and bond strengths to the teeth. *Biomaterials,* 23, 1819-29.

[97] Sideridou, I.; Tserki, V.; Papanastasiou, G. (2002). Effect of chemical structure on degree of conversion in light-cured dimethacrylate-based dental resins. *Biomaterials,* 23, 1819-29.

[98] Van Landuyt, K.L.; Snauwaert, J.; De Munck, J.; Peumans, M.; Yoshida, Y.; Poitevin, A,.; Coutinho, E.; Suzuki, K.; Lambrechts, P.; Van Meerbeek, B. (2007). Systematic review of the chemical composition of contemporary dental adhesives. *Biomaterials,* 28, 3757-3785.

[99] Omura, I.; Yamauchi,J.; Nagase, Y.; Uemura, F.; (1985). *Adhesive Composition* , US patent No. 4,539,382 (to Kuraray Co.).

[100] Huang, C.-T.; Jefferies, S.R. (1989). *Adhese Composition Which Bonds to collagen and Calcium,* European Patent No. 321,683 B1 (to Dentsply Co).

[101] Nemcek, J. Roberts, T.A. (1989). Polymerisable Composition. *European Patent No.* 132,929 B1 (to ICI)

[102] Ruse, N.D.; Smith, D.C. (1991). Adhesion to bovine dentin-surface characterization. *J. Dent. Res.* 70, 1002-1008.

[103] Salz, U.; Burtscher, P.; Vogel, K., Moszner, N.; Rheinberger,V. (1997). New adhesive monomers for dental application, *Polym Prepr.* 38 (2) 143-4.

[104] Anbar, M.; St. John, G.A.; Scott, A.C.(1974). Organic polymeric polyphosphonates as potential preventive agents of dental caries: in vitro experiments. *J Dent Res,* 53, 867-878.

[105] Anbar, M.; Farley, E.P. (1974). Potential use of organic polyphosphonates as adhesive in restoration of teeth. *J Dent Res,* 53, 879-888.

[106] Farley, E.P.; Johnes, R.L.; Anbar, M. (1977). Improved adhesion of acrylic restorative materials to dental enamelby precoating with monomers containing phosphonate groups, *J Dent Res,* 56, 943-952.

[107] Moszner, N.; Zeuner, F.; Fischer, U.K.; Rheinberger, V. (1999). Monomers for adhesive polymers, 2. Synthesis and radical

polymerization of hydrolytically stable acrylic phosphonic acids. *Macromol Chem Phys* 200, 1062-7.

[108] Moszner, N.; Zeuner, F.; Fischer, U.K.; Rheinberger, V. (2001). Monomers for adhesive polymers, 3. *Synthesis, radical polymerization and adhesive properties of hydrolytically stable acrylic phosphonic acid monomers.*

[109] Salz, U.; Zimmermann, J.; Zeuner, F.; Moszner, N.(2004). Hydrolytically stable monomers for self-etching enamel-dentin adhesives. *Polym Prepr* 45 (2) 325.

[110] Kazantsev, O.A.; Shirshin, K.V; Sivokhin, AP.; Tel'nov, S.V.; Zhiganov, I.V.; Kuznetson, A,E.; Mironycheva, Y.L.(2003). Hydrolysis of 2-hydroxy methacrylate in concentrated aqueous solutions. *Russ J Appl Chem,* 76, 1296-8.

[111] Moszner, N.; Zeuner, F.; Angermann, J.; Fischer, U.K.; Rheinberger, V. (2003). Monomers for adhesive polymers, 4. Synthesis and radical polymerization of hydrolytically stable cross-linking monomers. *Macromol Mater Eng,* 288,621-8.

[112] Fuskshima, T.; Itoh, T.; Inoue, Y.; Kawagushi, M.; Miazaki, K. (1999). Effect of dentin primers containing N-methylolacrylamide or N-methylolmethacrylamide on dentin pretreatment. *J Dent,* 27, 391-7.

[113] Hartmann, M.; Jacob, U.; Schulz, B.; Wermann, K.; (1982). Biozide Polymere. IV. Synthese und Polymerisation von Acylderivaten des N-Hydroxymethyl- und N-Aminomethyl-chloracetamids. *Acta Polym,* 33, 215-7.

[114] Moszner, N.; Angermann, J.; Rheinberger, V.; Zeuner, F. (2004). Dentalmaterialien auf der Basis von Hydroxyalkylacrylamiden. *Eur Pat,* 1,374,828 A1, Ivoclar Vivadent AG.

[115] Tagami, J.; Hosoda, H.; Imai,Y.; Masuhara, E. (1987). Evaluation of a new adhesive liner as an adhesive promoter and a desensitizer on hypersensitive dentin. *Dent Mater,* 6, 201-8.

[116] Itou, K.; Torii, Y.; Nishitani, Y.; Ishikawa, K.; Suzuki, K.; Inoue, K. (2000). Effect of self-etching primers containing N-acryloyl aspartic acid on dentin adhesion. *J Biomed Mater Res,* 51, 569-74.

[117] Torii, Y.; Itou, K.; Nishitani, Y.;Yoshiyama, M.; Ishikawa, K.; Suzuki, K.(2003). Effect of self-etching primers containing N-acryloyl aspartic acid on enamel adhesion. *Dent Mater,* 19, 253-8.

[118] Hecht, R.; Ludsteck, M. (2002). Initiator system for acidic dental formulations. *Ger Pat,* 1 0124 o29, 3M-ESPE AG.

[119] Antonucci, J.M.; Grams, C.L.; Termini, D.J. (1979). New initiator systems for dental resins based on ascorbic acid. *J Dent Res* 58, 1887-99.

[120] Nyunt, M.M.; Imai, Y.(1996). Adhesion to dentin with resin using sulfinic acid initiator system. *Dent Mater J,* 15, 175-82.

[121] Suh, B.; Feng, L.; Pashley, D.H. Tay, F.R. (2003). Factors contributing to the incompatibility between simplified-step adhesives and chemically cured or dual-cured composites. Part III. Effect of acidic resin monomers. 5, 267-82.

[122] Crivello, J.V.; Dietliker, K. Photoinitiators for free radical cationic and anionic photopolymerization. In: Bradley G, editor. *Surface coatings technology.* 2nd ed. New York: Wiley; 1998 p. 168ff.

Chapter 4

Applications of Polymers in Oral and Maxillofacial Surgery

Maxillofacial materials are used to correct facial defects resulting from cancer surgery, accidents or even congenital deformities. Noses, ears, eyes and orbits or any other part of the head and neck may be replaced by these prostheses. Maxillofacial prostheses are difficult to construct and have a relatively short life of six months to several years in service. They fail because of inherent problems with static and dynamic properties over varying periods and because of colour degradation. The prostheses are expensive to fabricate and many patients cannot afford frequent replacement.

Several types of materials are available for maxillofacial prostheses and they vary considerably in ease of preparation and physical properties.

Poly(methyl methacrylate) was once commonly used for maxillofacial prostheses and it is still used occasionally to make artificial facial parts. When properly pigmented, these prostheses can look quite realistic. The main disadvantages are that the acrylic is hard and heavy, does not flex when the face moves and does not have the feel of skin. Stone moulds are generally used with poly(methyl methacrylate) and these are sacrified when the prosthesis is deflasked after processing [1].

Resorbable sutures have many uses in oral and maxillofacial surgery to suture deep tissues. Catgut and collagen are used to elaborate natural resorbable sutures. Collagen is obtained from animal tendons; it is rarely used, although it seems to be less of an irritant than catgut. Submucous and serous layer of bovine intestine are used to elaborate catgut. This traditional material is a monofilamentary thread but exhibits a disadvantage: its diameter increases in only a few hours due to its absorption properties. Catgut can be simple or chromic. The latter is absorbed at a slower rate and is less of an irritant than simple catgut [2].

Poly(glycolic acid) (Figure 4.1) is a resorbable synthetic homopolymer. There are also copolymers of glycolic and lactic acid. *Polygluconates* and *Polydioxanone* are also employed as resorbable suture threads. Polygluconates are the salts of glyconic acid (Figure 4.1).

The tissue reaction produced against these synthetic materials is lower than that appearing for those of a natural origin. This is due to the different degradation processes involved in the resorption mechanism: physicochemical reactions for the polymers and enzymatic degradation for collagen and catgut. New materials for intra- and extraoral applications are appearing combining reduced tissue reaction with fast-absorbing properties. Among the nonresorbable threads, silk is the most used suture in oral and maxillofacial surgery. Capillary phenomena are its main disadvantage. Polyamides, polyester, polypropylene, polyacrylonitrile, etc., are also used as non-resorbable threads. All these threads tend to slacken slightly; thus more knots are required in order to tighten and reinforce the sutures [2].

Plasticized Polyvinylchloride has been used widely for maxillofacial applications, but it has been replaced by newer materials with superior properties. Polyvinylchloride is a rigid plastic with a glass transition temperature higher than room temperature. For maxillofacial applications, plasticizers are added to produce an elastomer at room temperature. Other ingredients added to polyvinylchloride include cross-linking agents for added strength and ultraviolet stabilizers for colour stability. There is no chemical reaction involved when the material is processed. The product is supplied as finely divided polyvinyl particles suspended in a solvent. When the fluid is heated above a critical temperature, the polyvinylchloride will dissolve in the solvent. When the mix is cooled an elastic solid is formed [1].

Polyurethane elastomers have great potential as maxillofacial materials. This hypothesis is based on their inherent environmental stability, high tear resistance, low modulus without the use of plasticizers, and good ultimate strength and elongation. They can accept intrinsic coloring and are amenable to maxillofacial processing techniques. Most importantly, the structure of the polyurethane polymer can be varied to optimize the desired properties and as a result polyurethanes are currently used in a variety of biomaterial applications.

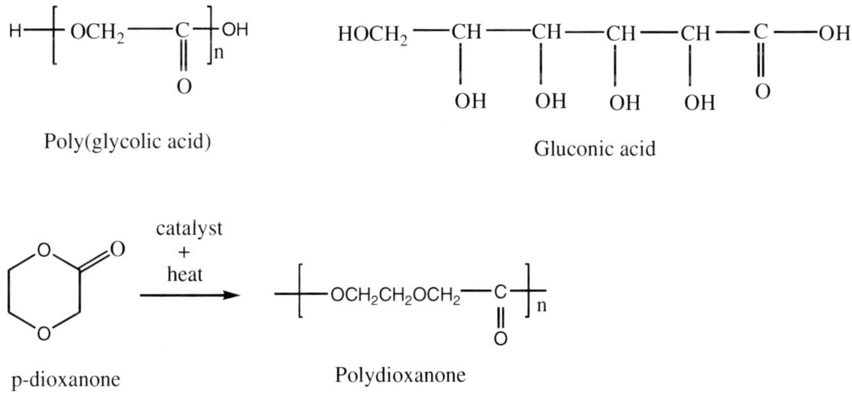

Figure 4.1. Chemical structure of poly(glycolic acid) gluconic acid and polydioxanone.

These polymers are formed by the reaction of diisocyanates and polyols (Figure 4.2). The former may be aromatic or aliphatic diisocyanates and the latter may be a di- or trifunctional polyether or a polyester macroglycol. The reaction may be accelerated by stannous octoate and must be conducted in the absence of moisture to avoid the formation of CO_2. Ultraviolet light stabilizers and antioxidants are mandatory for aromatic and advisable for aliphatic polyurethanes. Earth pigments are also used with these materials. Processing may be done in dry dental stone moulds at 273 K or in metal moulds. Since the reaction is stoichiometric, proportioning is critical as is the control of the processing temperature. The diisocyanates are very toxic and must be handled with extreme care [1].

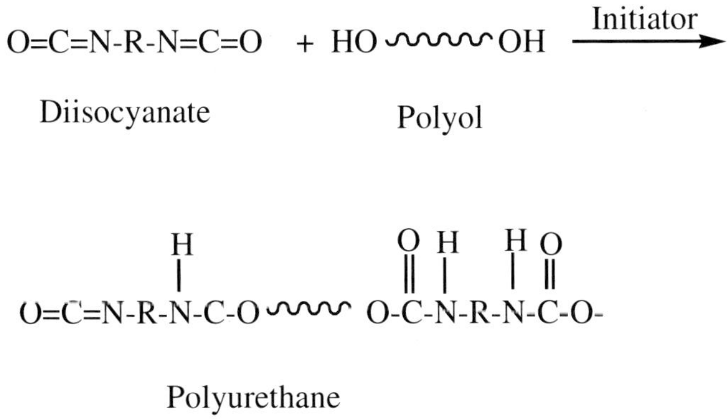

Figure 4.2. Synthesis of a polyurethane.

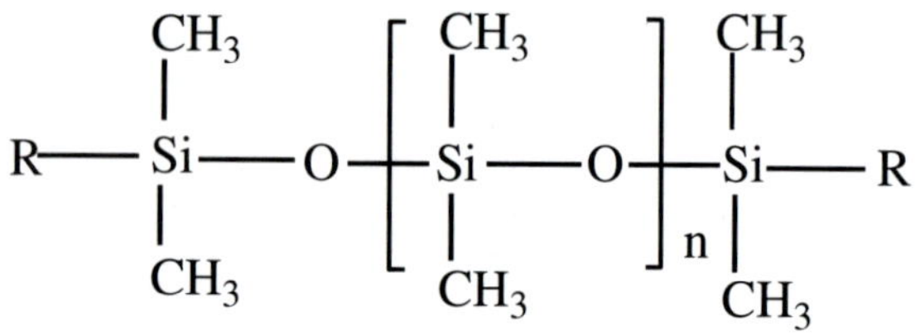

Polydimethylsiloxane

VARY n	*VARY R*
Higher n=more elastic	Hydroxy (OH)
ower n=more plastic	Vinyl ($CH=CH_2$)

Figure 4.3. Chemical structure of polydimethylsiloxane.

Silicon elastomers are the most widely used materials for maxillofacial prostheses. Silicone elastomers became commercially available in the late 1950s and remain the most commonly used to the present day, because they have good biocompatibility and biodurability, adequate mechanical properties and are easy to manipulate and mould.

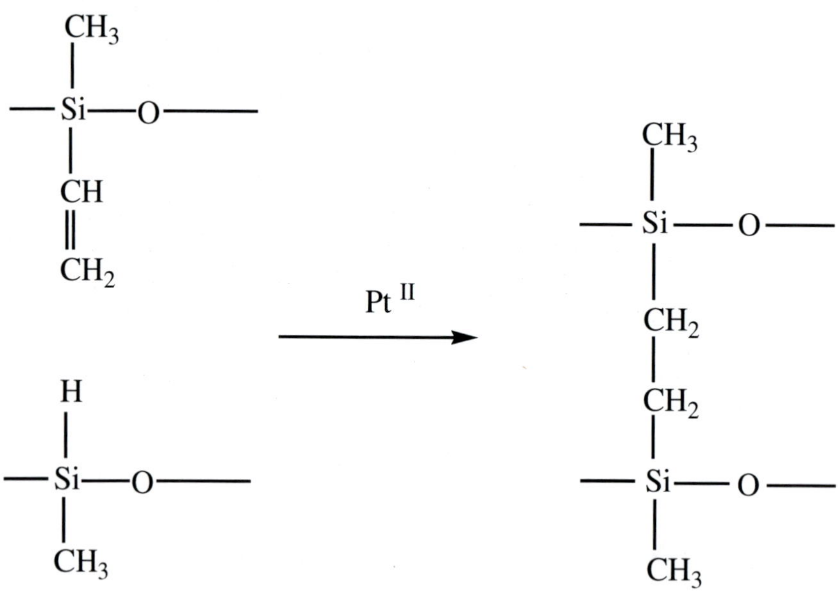

Figure 4.4. Cross-linking reaction between component A and component B.

The three most common silicones used for maxillofacial prostheses are Dow Corning MDX4-4210, Dow Corning Medical Adhesive Type A and Factor II, Inc.'s A-2186. The major components in A-2186 and MDX4-4210 are similar. Each is a pourable two-component silicone rubber and both materials cure by the same mechanism. The component A consists of a vinyl-terminated polydimethyl siloxane, reinforcing silica and a platinum catalyst. The component B (curing agent) consists of a hydrogen-terminated polydimethylsiloxane and an inhibitor. The crosslinking reactions between the two components are catalyzed by a platinum complex and involve the addition of silyl hydride groups (-SiH) of the component B to the vinyl groups (CH_2=CH-) of component A.

Although the materials have improved tear strength both A-2186 and MDX4-4210 have low adhesion to non-silicon based adhesives due to their hydrophobic nature. Because the curing reactions start immediately after the mixing of the two components, the working time of the materials is short.

Medical Adhesive Type A contains 10-20 wt% silica, 1-10 wt% $CH_3Si(OCOCH_3)_3$, 1-10 wt% methyltriacetoxysilane, 1-10 wt% ethyltriacetoxysilane, acetic acid (<1%) and stannous oleate (<1%). Upon application and exposure to moisture, the silane molecules are hydrolyzed by the water, which then undergo cross-linking reactions with the hydroxyl groups of the polysiloxane. The cross-linking reactions produce acetic acid as the by-product. Because Medical Adhesive Type A requires moisture to cure, the cure time is too long for curing the material inside a mould. Therefore, Medical Adhesive Type A is normally limited to use as a carrier for the extrinsic colorants applied to the surface of the prosthesis [3].

Materials proposed for maxillofacial applications should show high values of strength, toughness, and tear strength and low values of hardness and modulus. Tensile strength is a general measure of the overall strength characteristics of maxillofacial material. Although great strength is not always necessary, the minimum strength for clinical acceptance is difficult to be determined. Elongation is an indicator of the overall flexibility or "give" of a prosthetic material, and tear strength is indicative of the feathered edge and marginal integrity of the material in clinical service. Hardness is another measure of flexibility and reflects the "lifelike" quality of maxillofacial materials. Usually, the softer in materials more closely approximate the human skin. It has been that although the material must possess reasonable tensile strength, tear strength is assured. A high elongation necessarily means that much energy has to be dissipated before stress builds up sufficiently in the region of stress concentration to initiate and then propagate tearing. When a high elongation at the break is coupled with high tear strength, very satisfactory thin edge performance is assured [4].

4.1. LITERATURE

[1] Craig R.G. *Restorative Dental Materials.* St Louis, Missouri, Mosby-Year Book, Inc.

[2] Bascones, A.; Vega, J.M.; Olmo, N.; Turnay, J.; Gavilanes, J.G.; Lizarbe, M.A. Dental and Maxillofacial Surgery Applications of Polymers. In: Editor Severian Dumitriu. *Polymeric Biomaterials (Second Edition, Revised and Expanded).* New York: Marcel Dekker; 2001; 423-450.

[3] Lai, J.H.; Wang, L.L.; Ko, C.C.; DeLong, R.L.; Hodges, J.S. (2002). New Organosilicon maxillofacial prosthetic materials. *Dental Materials*, 18, 281-286.

[4] Polyzois, G.L. (1995). Evaluation of a new silicon elastomer for maxillofacial prostheses. *J Prosthod,* 4, 38-41.

Chapter 5

APPLICATIONS OF POLYMERS IN THERAPY OF GINGIVITIS AND PERIODONTITIS

Periodontal disease is a collective term ascribed to several pathological conditions characterized by degeneration and inflammation of gums periodontal ligaments, alveolar bone and dental cementum. It is a localized inflammatory response caused by bacterial infection of a periodontal disease, the expression of microbial pathogenic factors alone may not be sufficient to cause periodontitis. Periodontal pathogens produce harmful by-products and enzymes that break extracellular matrices as well as host cell membranes to produce nutrients for their growth. In doing so, they initiate damage directly or indirectly by triggering host-mediated responses that lead to self-injury.

In the early phase of the disease (gingivitis) inflammation is confined to the gingiva, but extends to deeper tissues in periodontitis , leading to gingival swelling, bleeding and bad breath. In the late phase of the disease, the supporting collagen of the periodontium is degenerated, alveolar bone begins to resorb and gingival epithelium migrates along the tooth surface forming a "periodontal pocket". This periodontal pocket provides ideal conditions for the proliferation of microorganisms. It however remains continues to harbor the bacteria associated with the disease, a potential for a further destructive phase exists. The disease may then require extensive treatment, failing which the teeth may be lost. Various stages of periodontitis are presented in Figure 5.1 [1].

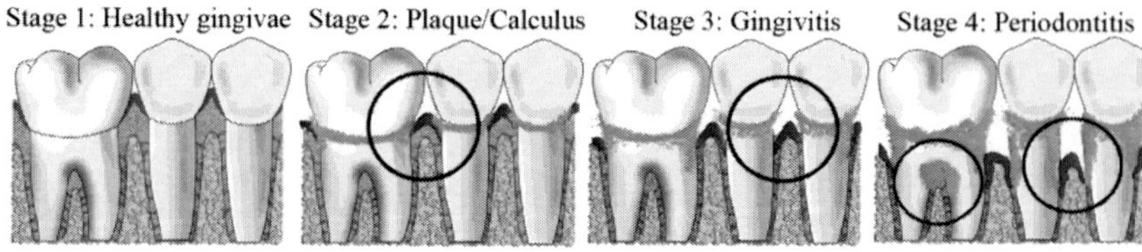

Figure 5.1. Diagrammatic representation of changes involved in the transition from healthy gingivae to the pathological periodontitis.

The applications of polymers in the therapy for gingivitis and periodontitis have evolved quite differently in these two areas, depending on the advancement made in the area of drug and polymer development and changes in patient populations and needs. The advancements that are most pertinent to polymers dealt with (1) their use as carriers for the controlled delivery of bioactive agents and particularly antimicrobials (2) their use in conjunction with tissue regeneration and healing and (3) factors pertinent to the effectiveness of implemented therapies [2].

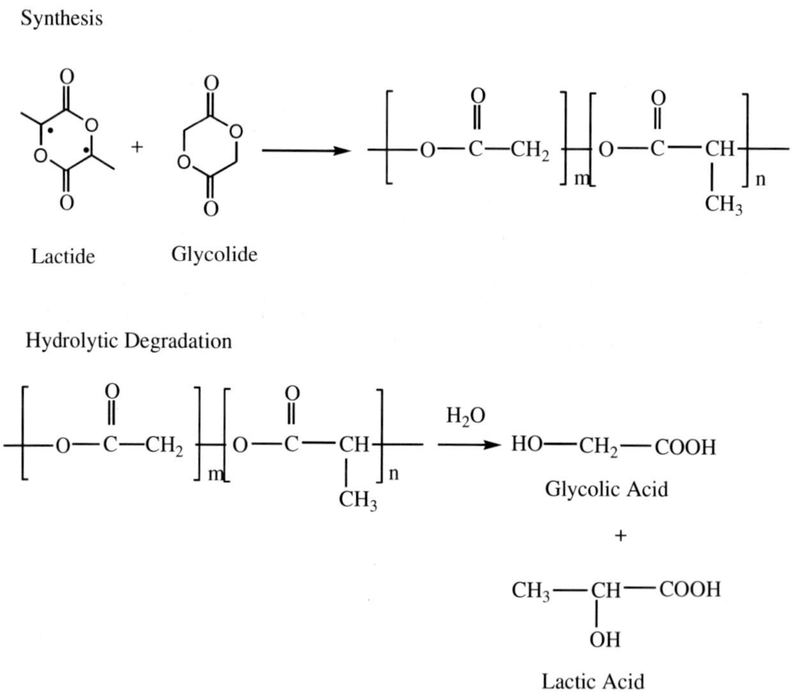

Figure 5.2. Synthesis and hydrolytic degradation of lactide-glycolide copolymer.

The use of systemic antibiotic for the treatment of periodontitis has shown some beneficial effect; however in recent years systemic antibiotics are only recommended for the treatment of rapidly progressing or refractory periodontitis. Multiple systemic doses of antibiotics have shown several drawbacks including inadequate antibiotic concentration at the site of the periodontal pocket, a rapid decline of the plasma antibiotic concentration to subtherapeutic levels, development of microbial resistance and high peak-plasma antibiotic concentrations, which may be associated with side effects. These obvious disadvantages have evoked an interest in the development of novel intra-pocket drug delivery systems for the treatment of periodontal disease. The periodontal pocket results from the progression of periodontal disease. The periodontal pocket provides a natural reservoir, which is easily accessible for the insertion of a delivery device. The gingival crevicular fluid provides a leaching medium for the release of a drug from the dosage form and for its distribution throughout the pocket. These features, together with the fact that the periodontal diseases are located to the immediate environment of the pocket, make the periodontal pocket a natural site for treatment with local delivery systems. Intra-pocket drug delivery systems are highly desirable due to the potentially lower incidence of undesirable side effects, improved efficacy and enhanced patient compliance. The attractiveness of treating periodontal diseases by the intra-pocket drug delivery systems is based on the prospects of maintaining effective high levels of drug in the gingival crevicular fluid for a prolonged period of time to produce the desirable clinical benefits [1].

5.1. Polymers for Controlled Drug Delivery

The majority of the early work on controlled delivery systems dealt with the administration of antimicrobials for the treatment of periodontitis and to a lesser extent, gingivitis. Early controlled delivery systems placed in or near the periodontal pocket or in the vicinity of a compromised gingival tissue consisted of (1) a reservoir-type device with a cellulose acetate dialysis tube (or hollow fiber) loaded with tetracycline, (2) monolithic fibers of ethylene vinyl acetate copolymer (EVA) and tetracycline , (3) a cellulose acetate dialysis tube containing chlorhexidine, (4) acrylic strips containing metronidazole, chlorhexidine or tetracycline, (5) an ethyl cellulose matrix containing chlorhexidine, (6) a collagen film containing chlorhexidine, (7) an injectable white petroleum gel loaded with tetracycline, chlorhexidine or stannous fluoride, (8) chlorhexidine or tetracycline in hydroxypropyl cellulose and (9) tetracycline or metronidazole in polyhydroxy butyric acid.

Phenomenal growth in the area of absorbable polymers over the past two decades affected significantly the dental community's approach to controlled drug delivery systems for use in the therapy for gingivitis and periodontitis. Absorbable polymers containing copolymers of lactide and glycolide and segmented copolymers of these monomers have played a key role in the development of several controlled drug delivery systems. The Scheme for the synthesis and degradation of a typical copolymer is shown in Figure 5.2.

Recent investigations dealing with the development of new drug delivery systems using polymeric materials as carriers are reviewed in reference [1] and [2].

5.2. Guided Tissue Regeneration

It is well established that progressive periodontitis leads to tooth loss through destruction of the tooth attachment apparatus. In teeth where continued function requires additional periodontal support, controlling the periodontal infection is not sufficient and regeneration of the lost periodontium is needed. Procedures used in the treatment of periodontal disease to achieve replacement or reconstitution of lost periodontal tissue have evolved over the past few decades and are denoted as regenerative therapy. Accordingly, periodontal regeneration is defined as restoration of lost supporting tissue, including new alveolar bone, cementum and periodontal ligament. New connective tissue attachment deals with the development of a new connective tissue with a root surface that has been deprived of its periodontal ligament, through the formation of new cementum by inserting collagen fibers. Guided tissue regeneration describes procedures designed to manipulate cells that repopulate the wound healing site leading to tissue regeneration [2].

Application of polymeric membranes in guided tissue regeneration evolved homopolymers or copolymers of polyglycolide and/or polylactide. Occlusive bioresorbable membranes made of polylactic or polyglycolic acid are equally successful as expanded polytetrafluoroethylene membranes in regenerating bone in transosseous defects in the rabbit mandibular ramus. One apparent advantage of poly(α-hydroxy acids) is their degradation by hydrolysis, resulting in decomposition products that are mostly metabolized to carbon dioxide and water. The degradation rate is dependent on the presence of enzymes, bacteria (infection) mechanical strain and pH. The addition of D-lactide or glycolide results in a faster degradation. However, the hydrolysis of these polymers releases lactic and/or glycolic acids; if the concentration of these monomers goes over a certain threshold they may be toxic to cells and present osteolytic effects [3].

5.3. LITERATURE

[1] Jain, N.; Jain, G.K.; Javed, S.; Iqbal, Zeenat, Talegaonkar, S.; Ahmad, F.J.; Khar, R.K. (2008). Recent approaches for the treatment of periodontitis. *Drug Discovery Today*, 13, 932-943.

[2] Shalaby, S, W.; Salz, U. Application of Polymers in the Therapy of Gingivitis, Periodontitis, and Treatment of dry Socket. In: Editor Shalaby, S. W. and Salz, U. *Polymers for Dental and Orthopedic Applications*. Boca Raton: Taylor and Francis Group; 2007; 145-163.

[3] Bascones, A.; Vega, J.M.; Olmo, N.; Turnay, J.; Gavilanes, J.G.; Lizarbe, M.A. Dental and Maxillofacial Surgery Applications of Polymers. In: Editor Severian Dumitriu. *Polymeric Biomaterials (Second Edition, Revised and Expanded)*. New York: Marcel Dekker; 2001; 423-450.

Chapter 6

APPLICATIONS OF POLYMERS IN ORTHODONTIC TREATMENTS

Orthodontics is a specialized field of dentistry that involves the application of mechanical forces to urge poorly positioned or crooked teeth into correct alignment and orientation. Orthodontic procedures can be used for cosmetic enhancement of teeth, as well as medically necessary movement of teeth to correct underbites or overbites. For example, orthodontic treatment can improve the patient's occlusion or enhanced spatial matching of the corresponding teeth.

The most common form of orthodontic treatment involves the use of orthodontic brackets and arch wires, which together are commonly referred to as "braces". Orthodontic brackets, more particularly the orthodontic bases are small slotted bodies configured for direct attachment to bands which are in turn cemented or otherwise secured around the teeth. Once the brackets are affixed to the patient's teeth, such as by means of glue or cement a curved archwire is inserted into the slot of each bracket. The arch wire acts as a template or track to guide movement of the teeth into proper alignment. End sections of archwire are typically captured within tiny appliances known as "buccal tubes" affixed to the patient's molar [1].

Conventional brackets requiring ligatures and self-ligating brackets have been formed from a wide variety of materials, including metal, plastic or a combination thereof. Eliades Theodore in a special article developed the current status of brackets and arch wires along with a projection of future developments in materials technology and clinical applications [2]. J. S. Russell in his recent article presents the currently available plastic and ceramic brackets and discusses the potential problems associated with each [3]. Recent advances, introduced by manufacturers in an attempt to overcome their clinical disadvantages, are described. Plastic brackets were first marketed in the early 1970's. Initially constructed from acrylic and later polycarbonate, polymer having functional groups linked together by carbonate groups –O-(C=O)-O- in a long molecular chain. However their acceptance by orthodontics as an aesthetic alternative to metal brackets was short lived. Inherent problems were soon noticed, including staining and odors but more importantly their lack of strength and stiffness resulting in bonding problems, tie wing fractures [4] and permanent deformation. Permanent deformation, or creep, occurs when a material is subjected to a constant load over an extended period of time and is particular important for thermoplastic materials such as polycarbonate resins. Polycarbonate bracket slots distorted with time under a constant physiologic stress (2000gm.-mm) rendering them insufficiently strong to withstand longer treatment times or transmit torque [5]. In a simulated intra-oral situation Harzer et al. [6] reported significantly higher torque losses and lower torquing moments with polycarbonate brackets compared to metal brackets. They recommended that manufacturers should provide data on the distortion to be expected in polycarbonate brackets, which must be offset by additional torque, or that the bracket should be omitted from the technical specification. To compensate for the lack of strength and rigidity of the original polycarbonate brackets, high-grade medical polyurethane brackets and polycarbonate brackets reinforced with ceramic or fiberglass fillers and/or metal slots have been recently introduced and are becoming increasingly popular. Polycarbonate brackets with metal reinforced slots demonstrate significantly less creep than conventional polycarbonate brackets [7] although torque problems still exist. Approximately 15% loss in torque over 24 hours has been observed with both ceramic reinforced and metal lined polycarbonate brackets [8]. However, the performance of these brackets is significantly better than polycarbonate brackets and they probably have the potential to challenge ceramic brackets with future development. When comparing torque deformation characteristics of seven commercially available plastic brackets against stainless steel brackets, Sadat-Khonsari et al. [9] showed that metal slot reinforced brackets were subjected to the lowest degree of deformation, followed by pure polyurethane, pure polycarbonate and fiberglass reinforced polycarbonate brackets. Ceramic reinforced polycarbonate brackets showed the highest deformation under torque stresses. The addition of ceramic and fiberglass in the plastic brackets also failed to improve the torque stability of the polycarbonate brackets and pure polyurethane brackets showed no significant difference from pure polycarbonate at optimal torque. A comparison with stainless steel brackets illustrated that plastic brackets are only suited for clinical application if they have a metal slot. Self-ligating aesthetic brackets are a further recent development. Polycarbonate self-ligating brackets have been shown in vitro to generate significantly greater static and kinetic frictional forces than stainless steel self-ligating brackets but are comparable to conventional stainless steel brackets [10].

Recently the use of crystalline polymers in forming the orthodontic brackets results in brackets exhibiting increased durability and strength. Amorphous polymeric materials may be blended with the crystalline polymers to provide enhanced elasticity, flexibility and toughness. One example of a class of suitable crystalline polymers for use in forming orthodontic brackets is poly(arylether ketones) a specific example of which is PEEK. The basic unit of the poly(arylether ketone) sold under the trade name PEEK is as follows:

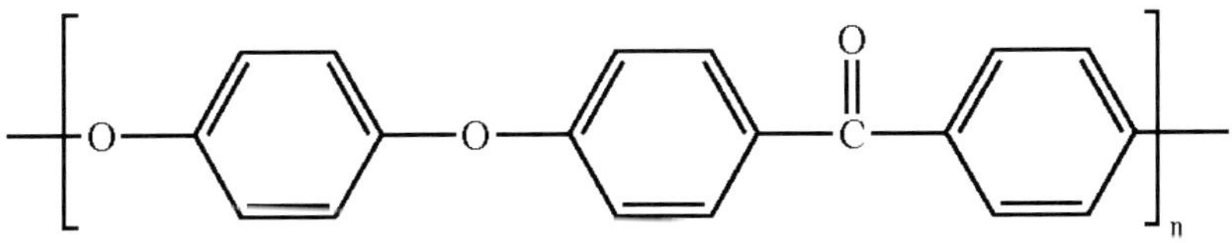

PEEK is a thermoplastic poly(arylether ketone) polymer that is capable of forming a crystalline structure that offers an outstanding combination of physical properties including excellent wear resistance, strength and stiffness.

Crystalline nylons are another class of suitable crystalline polymers for use in forming orthodontic brackets. A specific example of a crystalline nylon is Trogamid, manufactured by Degussa AG, located in Germany. The basic unit of one type of Trogamid nylon sold under the trade name Trogamid T is as follows:

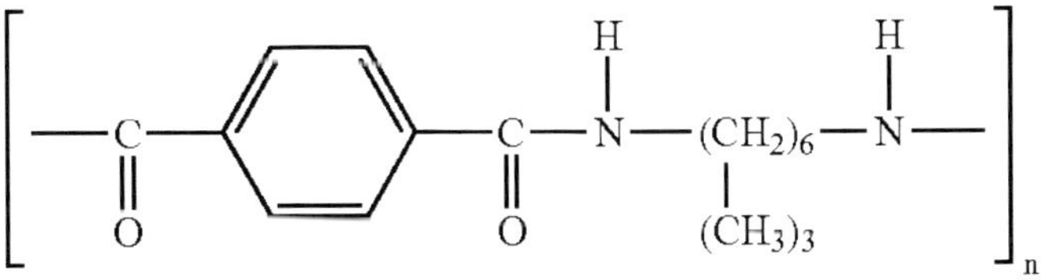

Trogamid is a thermoplastic polyamide polymer that is capable of forming a crystalline structure that offers an outstanding combination of physical properties including excellent wear resistance, strength and stiffness and transparency.

The orthodontic bracket may include an amorphous polymer. Examples of suitable amorphous polymeric materials include polyetherimides, a specific example of which is ULTEM, manufactured by General Electric. ULTEM polymers are amorphous and offer enhanced elasticity, flexibility and toughness at room temperature. Other suitable materials that could be used as an optional amorphous component include polycarbonate resins, amorphous poly(arylether ketone) resins, acetal polymer resins or other amorphous polymer resins known in the art [1].

Fiber reinforced composites are also currently being developed for use as orthodontic archwire materials. By adjusting the ceramic/polymer proportions, these wires can be manufactured in a wide range of clinically relevant levels of elastic stiffness, allowing practitioners to use variable-modulus orthodontic techniques without having to change arch wire materials as treatment progresses. Allergic reactions to nickel, which are a debatable concern for many metallic alloys are also averted with composite materials. With further developments in the near future fiber reinforced materials are expected to replace metals as the material of choice for orthodontic arch wires.

Fiber reinforced composite archwires for orthodontic purposes are fabricated using a procedure called pultrusion. Fiber bundles are pulled through an extruder in which they are wetted with a monomer resin. Next, the monomer is cured with heat and pressure resulting in polymerization. During curing the wetted fiber is formed into a desired cross-sectional morphology, which may be circular or rectangular. This wire may be also be further shaped into a different morphology by further curing, a process known as beta staging. For this, the monomer should initially only be partially cured. The volume percent of fiber in each composition may vary within a wide range, extending from as little as 5% to about 75-80%. With increasing amounts of fiber there will be an increase in the stiffness as well the yield strength of the material [11].

Recently the clinical application of a new fiber reinforced composite which incorporates S2 glass fibers in a Bis-GMA matrix has described. This is available in various configurations such as rope, woven strip and unidirectional strip. These materials are only partly polymerized during manufacture (pre-pregs) which makes them flexible, adaptable and easily contourable over the teeth. Later they are completed polymerized and can be bonded directly to the teeth. They can be applied for various purposes such as post treatment retention, as full arches or sectional arches and to renforce anchorage by joining teeth together. A particular advatage is that due to the direct bondability to teeth, they can obviate the need for brackets in specific situations. In addition they are highly esthetic and could thus be effective alternative to lingual appliances [l2].

Under- or overgrowth of one or both of the jaw bones can lead to reduced function and an unattractive facial appearance either of which may have lasting and significant psychosocial effects. Treatment of severe cases may require a combination of orthodontic appliances and orthognathic (corrective jaw) surgery. After surgery the cut bone needs to be immobilised to ensure that optimal healing takes place. Titanium plates used for fixation are recognised to be the "gold standard" but recent developments in biomaterials e.g. polylactic acid, polyglycolic acid and polydioxanone, have led to an increased usage of bioresorbable plates or screws for orthognathic surgery. The use of these biologically inert and resorbable plates for the fixation of facial bones in orthognathic surgery would appear to offer some clinical advantages over metal plates by eliminating the possible need for a second operation for their removal. However , whilst resorbable plates do appear to offer certain advantages over metal plates, concerns remain about the stability of fixation, the length of time required for their degradation and the possibility of foreign body reactions. Clinical complications which have been reported with certain of the polylactic acid and polyglycolic acid materials include inflammatory foreign body reactions, osteolysis around screws and delayed resorption. In addition a small number of material-related failures have been seen when these resorbable materials were used in bimaxillary procedures without postoperatve rigid intermaxillary fixation. Postoperative infection is another important complication which can occur with either system. Loose screws and wound dehiscene have been implicated, either of which may lead to plate exposure and subsequent early plate removal [13].

6.1. LITERATURE

[1] US 7,247,019 B2 Patent, 2007. Abels, N.; Backes, C-H. Orthodontic brackets made from polymeric materials that impart desired strength properties.

[2] Eliades, Th. 2007. Orthodontic materials research and applications: Part 2. Current status and projected future developments in materials and biocompatibility. *Am J Orthod Dentofacial Orthop, 131,*253-62.

[3] Russell J.S. 2005. Current Products and Practice Aesthetic Orthodontic Brackets. *Journal of Orthodontics*, *32*, 146-163.

[4] Arid JO, Durning P. 1987. Fractures of polycarbonate edgewise brackets. A clinical and SEM study. *Br J Orthod 14*, 191–5.

[5] Dobrin RJ, Kamel IL, Musich DR. 1975. Load-deformation characteristics of polycarbonate orthodontic brackets. *Am J Orthod , 67*, 24–33.

[6] Harzer W, Bourauel C, Gmyrek H. 2004. Torque capacity of metal and polycarbonate brackets with and without a metal slot. *Eur J Orthod 26*, 435–441.

[7] Alkire RG, Bagby MD, Gladwin MA, Kim H. 1997. Torsional creep of polycarbonate orthodontic brackets. *Dent Mater, 13*, 2–6.

[8] Feldner JC, Sarkar NK, Sheriden JJ, Lancaster DM. 1994. In vitro torque-deformation characteristics of polycarbonate brackets. Am J Orthod *Dentofac Orthop, 106*, 265–72.

[9] Sadat-Khonsari R, Moshtaghy A, Schelgel V, Kahl-Nieke B, Möller M, Bauss O. 2004. Torque deformation characteristics of plastic brackets: a comparative study. *J Orofac Orthop*, *65*, 26–33.

[10] Cacciafesta V, Sfondrini MF, Ricciardi A, Scribante A, Klersy C, Auricchio F. 2003. Evaluation of friction and stainless steel esthetic self-ligating brackets in various bracket-archwire combinations. *Am J Orthod Dentofac Orthop, 124*, 395–402.

[11] Valiathan, A.; Dhar, S. 2006. Fiber reinforced composite arch-wires in orthodontics: function meets esthetics. *Trends Biomater Artif Organs , 20, 16-19.*

[12] Burstone and A. Kuhlberg. 2000. Fiber-reinforced composites in orthodontics, *J Clin Orthod, 36* , pp. 271–279.

[13] Fedorowicz, Z.; Nasser, M.; Newton, T.; Oliver, R.; Resorbable versus titanium plates for orthognathic surgery. *Cochrane Database of Systematic Reviews*, Issue 4, 2008.

Chapter 7

POLYMERIC DENTAL IMPRESSION MATERIALS

An impression is a negative reproduction of a given area of the oral cavity. The area reproduced may be composed of either hard or soft tissues or both. The material must be inserted into the mouth while it is too soft to retain its shape. A rigid base is needed to carry it to the mouth and hold it against the tissues until it hardens. For this purpose, a variety of trays, called stock trays, are available. These are shaped to fit over the average maxillary and mandibular arches. Some can be trimmed and bent to the requirements of the individual patient. Trays may also be fabricated for each individual patient.

An impression material must meet a wide range of requirements in order to provide an accurate impression of the different tissues. The following are some of the more important requirements.

1. The material should flow or be pliable at a temperature that will not injure the oral tissue.
2. It should set quickly, preferably within 2 to 4 minutes, at body temperature.
3. It should unite into a solid mass without adhering to the oral tissues or to the material used for the cast.
4. It should fall into all irregularities and fine lines in the area to reproduce without displacing soft tissue.
5. It must retain an accurate reproduction of surface detail when it solidifies and is withdrawn from the mouth.

6. It must have dimensional stability. It must not expand, contract, or become deformed in any way because of temperature changes, atmospheric conditions, or the pouring of the cast.
7. It must not be too unpleasant to the patient.
8. It must not flake (after solidifying) when trimmed with a sharp knife at room temperature.

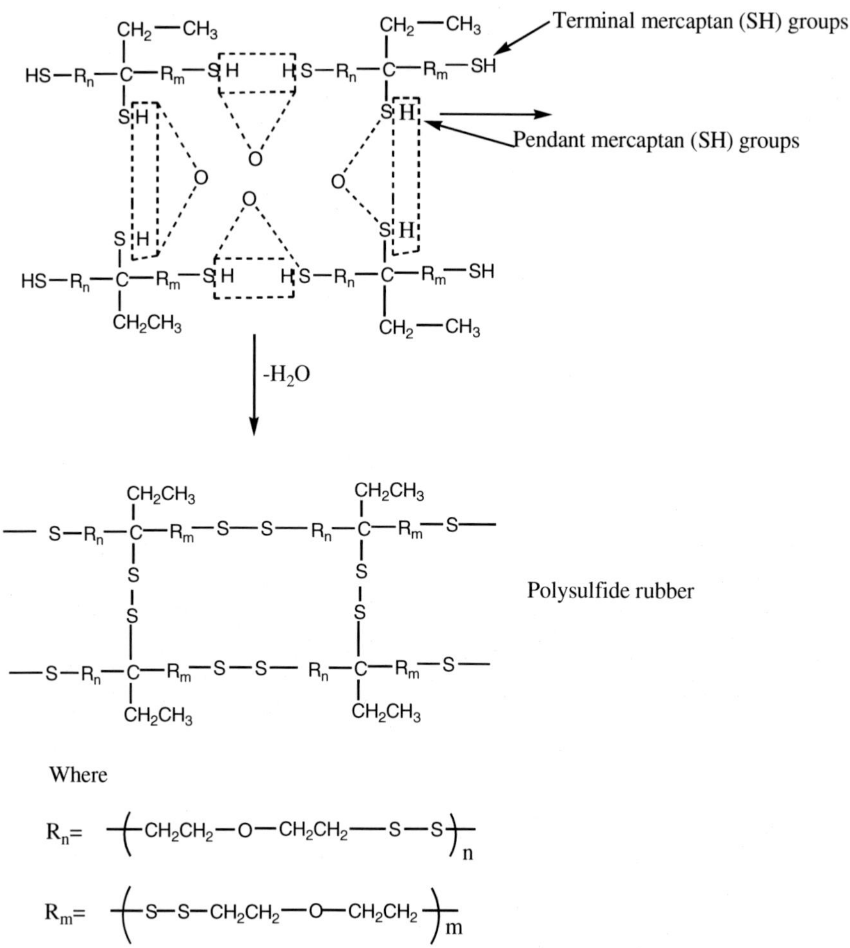

Figure 7.1. Setting reaction of a polysulfide impression materials.

Impression materials are of three types: the rigid type, the thermoplastic type, and the elastic type. Thermoplastic materials soften when warmed and harden when cooled with no change in chemical makeup. Elastic materials expand and contract with no change in structure or shape. All three types have advantages and disadvantages. The dental officer determines which material best meets the requirements of each particular case. He frequently will use two or more materials to make a single impression.

Synthetic rubber base impression materials are flexible, rubber-like, and sufficiently elastic to return to their original shape after slight distortion. They are used for making impressions of areas containing undercuts, especially for crowns, inlays, and removable and fixed partial dentures. There are three types of rubber base impression materials. Type one has a synthetic rubber base of polysulfide. Type two has a synthetic rubber base of silicone and type three has a synthetic rubber base of polyether. All types are polymeric compounds [1-5].

7.1. POLYSULFIDES

Polysulfide impression materials are supplied as two pastes in collapsible tubes, one labeled "base" and the other labeled "accelerator" or "catalyst". The ingredients of a typical polysulfide rubber impression material are: polysulfide 80-85 wt% and titanium dioxide, zinc sulfate, copper carbonate or silica 16-18 wt% for the base and lead dioxide 60-68 wt%, dibutyl or octyl phthalate 30-35 wt% (plasticizers used to form a paste of the correct consistency) sulfur 3 wt% and other substances such as magnesium stearate and deodorants 2 wt% for the accelerator. The base paste is usually colored white because of the color of the filler, while the accelerator paste is brown colored due to the lead dioxide. The polysulfide has a molecular weight of 2000 to 4000 and contains three –SH groups; two of these groups are terminal and one is pendant. The terminal and pendant groups of adjacent molecules are oxidized by the accelerator to produce chain extension and cross-linking respectively (Figure 7.1)

The reaction causes a rapid increase of molecular weight, and the mixed paste is converted to a rubber. Although the mixes set to a rubber in about 10 to 20 minutes, polymerization continues and the properties change for a number of hours after the material sets. Cross-linking is used to reduce the permament deformation (increase the recovery) of the set rubber under compression or extension during removal from the mouth. The ingrendients and their weight per cent may vary from one product to another. In general, the weight percent of the filler in the base paste increases from low to medium to high consistencies. Although the most common active ingredient in the accelerator is lead dioxide, some magnesium oxide may also be present. Whitening agents cannot cover the dark color of the lead dioxide; thus these pastes are dark brown to grey-brown in colour.

Properties of clinical interest are (1) toxicity (2) colour of the base and accelerator (3) time required for mixing (4) working time (5) consistency (6) permament deformation during removal (7) dimensional stability (8) flow after setting (9) flexibility (10) reproduction of detail (11) compatibility with die and model materials and (12) deterioration during storage of the unmixed material. Although most of the accelerator pastes contain lead dioxide, when the materials are used as directed they have been shown to have no toxic effects. Ain general the working time for polysulfide rubber impression materials decreases as the consistency becomes stiffer (light to heavy bodied). The working time is an indication of the maximum time allowed before the impression time allowed before the impression material should be in the mouth with typical values being 5 to 7 minutes. The final setting time is usually in the range of 8 to 12 minutes from the start of mixing.The permanent deformation values of 2% to 3% (97% to 98% recovery) obtained when the material is held under 12% compression for 30 seconds indicate that the polysulfides are not perfectly elastic and that compression during removal of the impression material should be kept to a minimum. Polysulfide rubber provides excellent reproduction of surface detail and is readilty capable of reproducing fine lines 0.025 mm wide.The polysulfide materials have excellent shelf life but should not be stored in a warm location; the tubes should be checked to determine if the caps are on tightly before they are stored. One can extend the shelf life by storing unused material in the refrigerator. It should be emphasized that the strength and permament deformation properties of the polysulfide materials continue to improve for several hours after they are set. Several minutes extra in the mouth results in noticeable improvement; however the time in the mouth has a practical limitation.

The advantages of polysulfide impression materials are:

a) Acceptable dimensional stability, which was only bettered with the advent of the addition silicon materials.
b) The highest strength of all impression materials.
c) The disadvantages are :

d) They are rather slow setting
e) Their permanent set is inferior to all types of silicon polymers, except those which are heavily loaded with filler
f) Not surprisingly they are rather odiferous materials that are rather messy to handle

Alternatives reactors to PbO_2 have been tried, for example cumene hydroperoxide or t-butyl hydroperoxide. However these constituents are volatile and its loss by evaporation leads to shrinkage of the set mass. Another development replaced the PbO_2 by a zinc carbonate/organic accelerator system.

7.2. SILICONES

The impetus for the development of silicon impression materials resulted from several criticisms of the polysulfide materials, such as their objectionable odor, the staining of linen and unuiforms by the lead dioxide, the amount of effort required to mix the base with the accelerator, the rather long setting times, the moderately high shrinkage on setting and the fairly high permament deformation.Two types of silicones are used as impression materials: (1) condensation and (2) addition (some times called "vinyl silicon") types. The names identify the type of polymerization reaction.

7.2.1. Condensation Type

The material is supplied as a base and an accelerator or catalyst.The base paste contains a moderately low-molecular weight silicon liquid called a dimethyl siloxane, which has reactive OH groups (Figure 7.2). The accelerator may be a liquid that consists of stannous octoate suspension and alkyl silicate, or it may be supplied as a paste by adding a thickening agent. The reaction proceeds as mentioned producing a three dimensional network rubber with the liberation of ethyl alcohol and an exothermic temperature rise of about $1^{o}C$.

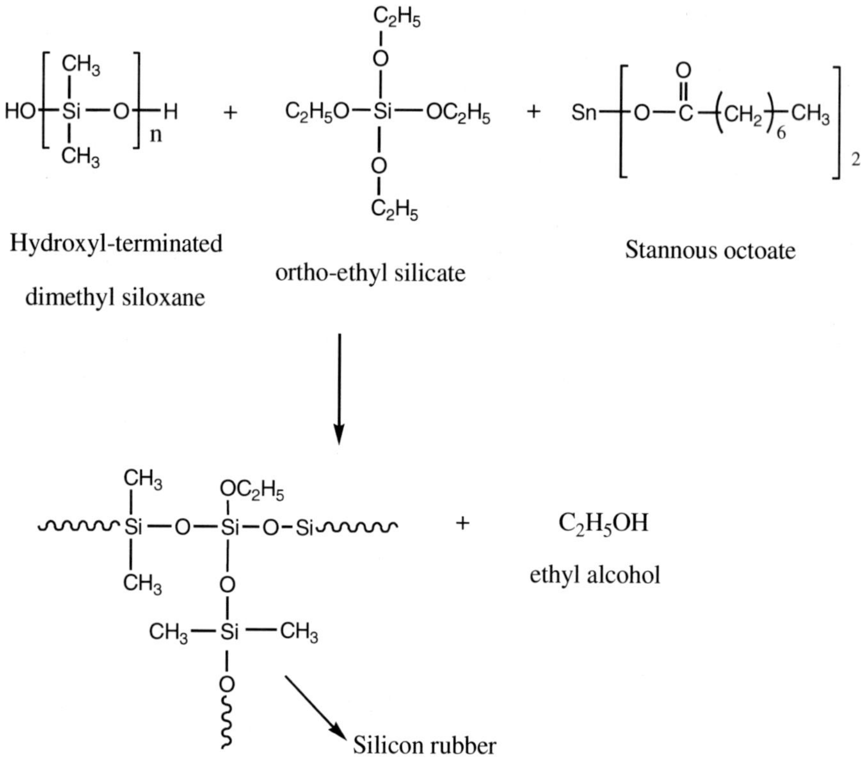

Figure 7.2. Condensation reactions in silicon rubber formation.

The silicon pastes are supplied in light-, regular- and heavy-bodied consistencies as well as a very heavy consistency called a “putty” The consistency is controlled by the selection of the molecular weight of the dimethylsiloxane and the concentration of the reinforcing agent. Higher molecular weights are used with the heavier-bodied materials. The concentration of the reinforcing agent increases from 35% for light-bodied consistency to 75% for the putty consistency. The polymerization accompanied by the release of the byproduct causes a shrinkage that is greater in the low consistency than in putty like consistency. The accelerator does not have unlimited shelf life because the stannous octoate may oxidize and the ortho-ethyl silicate is not entirely stable in the presence of the tin ester.

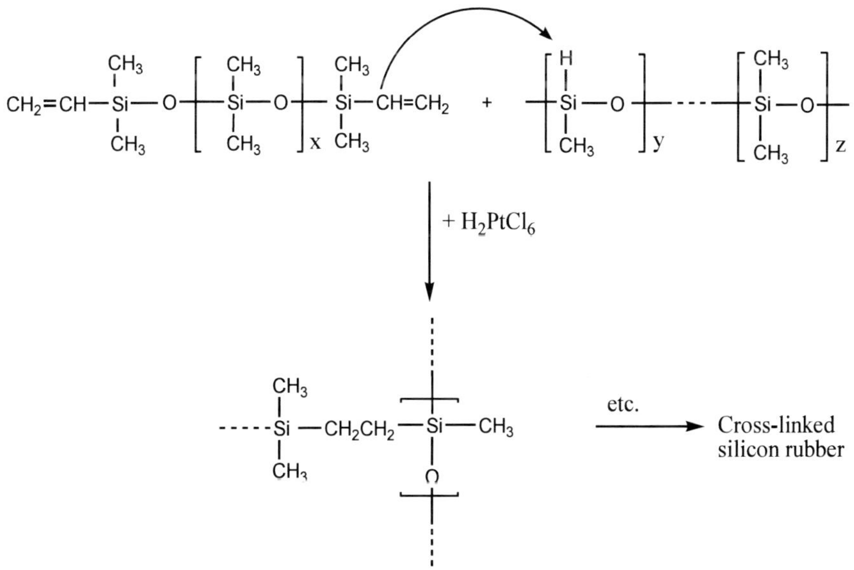

Figure 7.3. Simplified form of the reaction for preparation of a cross-linked silicon rubber of addition type.

7.2.2. Addition Type

The material is supplied as a two paste or a two-putty system with one containing a low-molecular weight silicon having terminal vinyl groups, reinforcing filler and a chloroplatinic acid catalyst and the other containing a low-molecular weight silicon having silanes hydrogens and reinforcing filler. The two are mixed in equal quantities and the addition reaction occurs between the vinyl and hydrogen groups with no by-product being formed. A simplified setting reaction is as follows:

The vinyl soloxane is difunctional and the hydrogen-containing siloxane is multifunctional. No volatile by product is formed in this reaction and minimal dimensional change occurs during polymerization. Increases in temperature increase the rate of reaction and shorten the setting time.

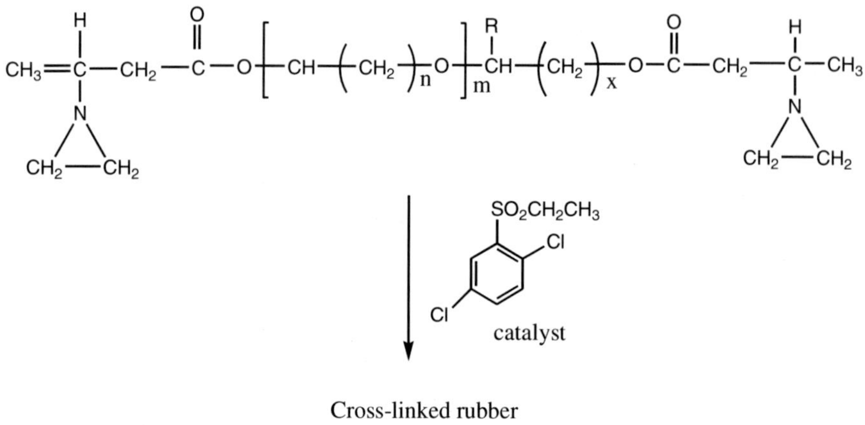

Figure 7.4. Simplified form of the reaction for preparation of a polyether.

7.3. POLYETHERS

Polyether systems offer the possible combination of mechanical properties better than those of polysulfides along with less dimensional change than those of condensation silicone impression materials. They are also hydrophilic and have good wetting properties. They have limiting features such as short working time and high stiffness. Polyether rubber impression materials are supplied as a base and catalyst system. The base is a moderately low-molecular weight polyether, containing ethylene imine terminal groups. These terminal groups are reacted together by the action of an aromatic sulfonic acid ester catalyst to form a cross-linked high molecular rubber as illustrated in Figure 7.3.

A silica filler is incorporated in the base as well as a plasticizer such as glycol ether phthalate. The catalyst paste contains 2,5-dichlorobenzene sulfonate, as a cross-linking agent, along with a thickening agent. A separate tube contains a thinner that includes octyl phthalate and about 5% methyl cellulose as a thickening agent. Coloring agents may be addede to base and accelerating as desired. A polyether system is also supplied as low- and high-viscosity types.The reaction in a simplified form is shown in Figure 7.4. The rubber is formed by cationic polymerization and opening of the imine rings. The backbone of the polymer is believed to be a copolymer of tetrahydro furan and ethylene oxide. The setting reaction is slightly more exothermic than that of other rubber impression materials, with a temperature rise of about 4°C.

7.4. LITERATURE

[1] Combe, E.C.; Burke, F.J.T; Douglas, W.H. *Dental Biomaterials.* Boston: Kluwer Academic Publishers; 1999.

[2] Craig, R.G. *Restorative Dental Materials.* 10th ed. St Louis, Missouri: Mosby-Year book, Inc. 1997.

[3] Van Noort, R. *Introduction to Dental Materials.* 2nd ed. Edinburgh: Mosby, 2002.

[4] Braden, M.; Clarke, R.L.; Nicholson, J.; Parker, S. *Polymeric Dental Materials.* Berlin Heidelberg: Springer-Verlag 1997.

INDEX

B

C

D

E

F

G

H

I

J

K

L

M

N

O

Q

R

T

U

V

W

X

Y

Z